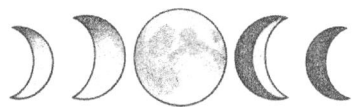

Diary of a Luteal Fugitive

A True Story of PMDD

PUBLISHED BY: Jo Grey

I wake up already wrong.

The duvet feels too heavy. The light through the curtains too sharp. My chest, tight. My limbs, electric and dead all at once. Something is coming. Or maybe it's already here.

I shuffle to the bathroom, avoid the mirror. I can't look today. My own face feels like a stranger's. My body feels poisoned with something I can't name. I brush my teeth too hard. I gag. I want to scream. But instead, I spit and rinse and try not to cry this early in the day.

Nothing has happened. And yet, everything is wrong.

A text pings. I don't read it. It's from someone who loves me, but today that feels like an accusation. I stare at it until it fades from the lockscreen. A tiny silence. A tiny shame.

My brain starts lying, fast, cruel lies that sound like truth.
You're too much.
You're broken.
No one could love this version of you.
You're dangerous.

I believe every word.

By 9am, I've snapped at someone I love. By 11, I've planned my exit from life in exquisite detail. By 2, I've forgotten how to feel anything but dread.

This is not a bad mood. This is a chemical war.

And it happens every month.

Half a life stolen, month by month, year by year, and no one taught me the name for it until I was already bleeding.

But you're here now.
And maybe this time, we'll name the storm before it hits.

Contents

PART

One

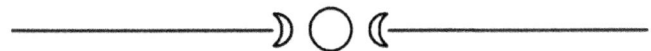

The Disappearance

1.1 Where Did I Go?

The terrifying experience of vanishing into yourself

There's a moment, maybe it's a brief flicker or maybe it's a landslide, when I feel myself disappear. Not physically. Not in a way you'd notice from the outside. But inside, something quietly folds in on itself. It's like my inner self, my soul, my *self*, just steps back, or sinks, or switches off. And someone else, something else, takes my place.

I've stood in front of a mirror and not recognised my own eyes. They looked back at me, wide and hollow, ringed with exhaustion and thick with a sadness I didn't understand. Sometimes they were angry, wild. Sometimes they were blank. But never mine. I stared and whispered, *Where did I go?*,and I didn't have an answer.

People talk about "mood swings" like they're some cute little pendulum. A little cranky. A little weepy. A day of chocolate and tissues. But this is not that. PMDD is not a mood. It's an unmaking.

There are days I wake up and I already know she's here. The other me. The Luteal Me. I feel it in my chest first. Like a heaviness that settles before I've even opened my eyes. Before I've had a thought. Before I've had a chance to fight. That's how early she starts.

And when she's here, I vanish.

I don't mean metaphorically. I mean: the things I like? Gone. The way I speak? Gone. The softness in my laugh, the way I reach for people, the little sparkle I carry when I'm whole, gone, gone, gone. In its place: flatness. Or rage. Or deep, wet grief. Or numbness so complete I start wondering if I'm even real.

I've written texts that don't sound like me. I've deleted photos because I didn't want proof that I existed in that body, on that day. I've screamed at people I love and not remembered why. I've laid in the shower, shaking, trying to understand what I did wrong to deserve this cycle of self-erasure.

I didn't know, at first, that this had a name. It just felt like every month I went missing. Like being kidnapped by my own biology. Like time travel, but only to a version of myself I didn't want to meet. I would crash into myself like a wave, over and over. And then, when it was over, when the bleeding started, I'd float back into myself, blinking, confused, ashamed, and exhausted.

I'd clean up the mess she left behind.

The worst part? No one saw it happen. I wasn't bleeding. I wasn't bruised. I wasn't in a hospital. I looked fine. And that made it harder. Because how do you explain that you're *missing* when your body is right there?

PMDD lives in the dark. It hides in plain sight. It's a disappearing act that takes place beneath your skin. And it doesn't happen once. It happens *every single month*. For years. Sometimes decades. Can you imagine that? Knowing you're going to lose yourself, again and again, and there's nothing you can do to stop it?

The terror of that, of being *reliably unstable*, is something I wouldn't wish on anyone.

It's not just about the feelings. It's about the fear that you can't trust your own mind. It's about saying things and doing things that feel like they're being beamed through you from some other place. It's about losing access to logic, to patience, to love. It's about becoming a person you do not recognise, but who wears your face.

Some days, I would find myself crying over nothing. Not sad tears, existential ones. The kind of crying where your bones feel hollow and your breath gets stuck. Where you can't even name what's wrong, because it's *everything*. Other days, I'd snap like a brittle branch. I'd throw words like daggers, cut people down, burn bridges I didn't mean to set alight. And then I'd hate myself for it. Hate myself *so much* that I'd begin to wonder if I deserved to feel this way. If I was just a terrible person, full stop.

But I wasn't. I'm not.

That's the cruellest trick PMDD plays. It doesn't just make you suffer, it convinces you it's your fault. That you're somewhat broken. That you're dangerous. That the real you *is* the monster. That the part of you who smiles and dreams and plans and loves, that part's the illusion.

I clung to that lie for a long time.

It's hard to fight for yourself when you don't know who that self is anymore. It's hard to speak up when your words twist in your mouth. When you're articulate one week and barely functional the next. When you've forgotten birthdays, cancelled plans, ghosted friends. When you've quit jobs, ruined relationships, stopped writing, stopped painting, stopped laughing.

Where did I go?

I went underground.

I became a fugitive in my own life, hiding from the wreckage I caused, hiding from the people who didn't understand, hiding from the grief of losing myself, over and over again.

And when I did return, on those quiet, post-storm days of lucidity, I was raw. Hungover from myself. Trying to apologise for things I couldn't even explain. Trying to rebuild bridges with no tools. Trying to reassure people I was okay when I didn't believe it myself.

It's a lonely kind of suffering.

I'm telling this story now, out loud, in ink, on purpose, because if you've ever felt yourself disappearing too, I want you to know you're not alone. You're not crazy. You're not weak. And this thing that's eating your edges every month? It has a name. It's real.

And maybe that's the beginning. Not of a cure, but of a reckoning. A way to finally say: I am here. I was always here. Even when I vanished.

1.2 The Silent Performer

Smiling through breakdowns, faking normal

No one suspected a thing.

That's the performance of it. The great vanishing act. The act *within* the act. Because while my insides crumbled, my outside smiled. I laughed. I replied to emails. I clinked glasses at birthday dinners. I said "I'm good, just tired," with such easy charm you'd never think to question it. But I was unravelling. Quietly. Violently. Invisibly.

I became a master at playing myself.

It wasn't even intentional at first. It was survival. A desperate attempt to keep the mask in place because if I let it slip, even for a second, I was scared everything would come pouring out. And once it poured, who would stay?

So of course I smiled. Through panic attacks. Through rage. Through the thick fog of disconnection. Through the deep, bone-heavy ache of depression that sat on my chest like a lead blanket.

Some days I would stare at my phone, heart racing, while I typed cheerful replies I didn't feel. "Haha omg YES," I'd send. Or "Totally fine! Just busy" when in reality, I'd spent the last hour curled into a ball on the bathroom floor, trying not to scream. Then I'd open the door, splash cold water on my face, and go back to being Her, the girl everyone expected me to be.

I went to work with a straight spine and a polite smile, even when my thoughts were static and my body felt like it didn't belong to me. I took calls. I made jokes. I replied to messages like I wasn't fraying at the edges. No one saw me flinch under fluorescent lights, or grip my own hands in meetings to stop them shaking. No one saw me cry in the toilet cubicle between clients, wipe it away, and walk back out like nothing happened.

I could perform "okay" with such conviction, even I almost believed it. Almost.

But my body always knew the truth.

It trembled when I held too much in. It broke out in rashes. My jaw ached from clenching. My digestion went wild. My sleep came in broken patches. And still, I smiled. I worked. I kept the world turning. Because PMDD doesn't pause your responsibilities. It just makes them harder. Heavier. Harsher.

There were days I'd be mid-conversation with someone and feel the tears rise in my throat like bile. But I'd swallow them. Nod. Laugh. Finish the sentence. Then go somewhere private and fall apart.

I've sat through dinners where every sound felt too loud, every light too bright, every word from someone else like an alien language I was supposed to decode. But I'd raise my glass, toast the moment, tell a funny story. I'd bite the inside of my cheek just to stay grounded. I'd rehearse what "normal" looked like and copy it beat for beat.

If you've never experienced it, it's hard to explain what it takes to pretend to be okay when your mind is at war with itself.

It's not just exhausting. It's annihilating.

Because you begin to believe that you can't show the truth. That the truth is *too much*. That your feelings will drive people away. That your darkness is a burden to others. That if you let people see the real you, this broken, bleeding, raging version, they'll stop loving you. Or worse, they'll look at you with pity instead of care.

So, you act. And act. And act. Until it doesn't even feel like acting anymore. It just feels like *you*. Or the you that the world is allowed to see.

But inside? You're gone.

You start losing access to your own truth. Your own voice. You stop asking for help. You downplay your symptoms. You lie. You say "It's not that bad," even when it is. You say "I'm just being dramatic," even when you're drowning. You turn into a perfectly pleasant hologram, floating through your life, saying all the right things at the right times, while screaming silently beneath the surface.

And the worst part is: you get praised for it.

"You're always so strong."
"You're so good at holding it all together."
"You seem so grounded."

Compliments that sound like kindness but feel like pressure. Pressure to *keep performing*. To not let the cracks show. To be everyone's favourite version of yourself, even when it's killing you.

There were times I'd look around a room full of people and think, *If I told you what's really going on inside me right now, you'd never look at me the same.*

So, I didn't tell them.

I performed instead.

No one clapped at the end of the show. Because there was no end. Just blackout curtains, and then another day. Another act. Another month.

Sometimes, I'd try to hint. I'd say things like, "I've been a bit off lately," or "I'm really struggling with my cycle," or "I don't feel like myself." But people would nod politely, unaware that I was hanging by a thread. That behind those casual words was a desperate plea: *Please notice. Please help. Please see me.*

PMDD doesn't come with a cast. It doesn't leave visible bruises. It doesn't get sympathy cards or casseroles. It just… exists in the shadows. And so you keep it there. Quiet. Hidden. Polished.

I think one of the most dangerous things about PMDD is how *good* we get at faking wellness. How the world teaches us to be palatable, agreeable, tidy. How we contort our pain into something acceptable, something that won't make other people uncomfortable.

But I am done performing.

I want to be messy. Honest. Human. I want to say, *I'm not okay*, and not feel like I'm failing. I want to be seen in my truth, in my hormonal chaos, in my darkness, and still be held.

Because performing might make you look strong, but it makes you feel invisible.

And I'm not invisible.

I'm here. And this is me. Raw. Real. Mid-breakdown. Mid-healing. Mid-story.

And I'm not smiling to make you feel better anymore.

1.3 The Ghost in the Mirror

Reconnecting (or failing to) with the 'real' self

She looks like me but I can tell
she's living in a private hell.
The eyes are mine but cracked with pain,
she smiles like she's not quite sane.

She talks like me but sounds too flat,
like she forgot where she was at.
Her laugh is wrong, her hands are slow,
she's someone I don't really know.

I touch the glass. She doesn't move.
I try to speak, to find some proof.
But silence pools inside her face,
I'm staring into empty space.

Sometimes I look in the mirror and don't know who I'm looking at. The reflection blinks, breathes, tilts its head just like me. But the eyes are distant. Like they belong to someone else entirely. Not a stranger. Not an enemy. Just... a ghost. A faded version of someone I used to be.

This is the part that's hardest to explain. It's not just the mood swings or the rage or the exhaustion. It's the slow disintegration of identity. The feeling that I am being peeled away from myself.

When I'm in the thick of PMDD, the "real" me feels like a memory. She's quiet. Too far away to touch. I try to summon her. I beg her to come back. But the connection is loose. Slippery. I feel like I'm reaching through fog for a face I used to wear.

I remember her. I remember how she laughed. How she got excited about books and silly memes and little plans. I remember her energy. The ease in her shoulders. The steadiness in her eyes. But when PMDD descends, that version of me evaporates. She doesn't feel real anymore. She becomes a story I once told myself. A character in a play that got cancelled halfway through.

And what's left behind is someone I barely recognise.

I go through the motions. Shower. Eat something. Answer a message. Smile when required. But underneath it all, I feel like I'm made of glass. Brittle. Hollow. Waiting to crack. I watch myself in the mirror and think, "That isn't me." I look tired in a way makeup can't fix. There's a dullness in my skin. A sadness in my posture. Sometimes, I try to mimic my old expressions, as if I can trick myself into feeling normal. I pull up my cheeks into a smile and try to hold it. But it never reaches my eyes. It feels like wearing a mask that doesn't quite fit.

I start talking to myself like a lost lover. Quietly, in my head. "Come back," I whisper. "Please. I miss you." But I don't always know who I'm talking to. Or if she's even still in here.

I want to say this gently, but I need to say it honestly: this loss of self is violent. It erodes you. It makes you doubt every part of who you are. Your choices. Your voice. Your memories. I have days where I can't trust anything I think. I look at my own reflection and feel like I'm impersonating someone. I keep searching for the person I used to be before the cycle swallowed her whole.

When the PMDD wave passes, I often don't feel relief. I feel grief. Because I realise how far away I went. How long I was gone. How much I missed. I start counting the damage. The things I said. The things I cancelled. The way I went cold or cruel or disappeared from people's lives, even if only for a few days. The apologies stack up. The shame does too.

Reconnecting with myself is not like flicking a switch. It's more like finding my way home through rubble. I pick through the mess, looking for pieces of me that survived. A song I still like. A joke that still makes me laugh. The feel of sunlight on my face and the moment I realise I can actually feel it again. Not just see it. Not just pretend to appreciate it. But truly feel it.

Some months, the reconnection happens faster. A morning arrives and I feel it in my chest. The weight has lifted. My brain is clearer. I make a coffee and something in me softens. I remember what peace feels like. I remember what *I* feel like. It's like being welcomed back into my own body.

Other months, it takes longer. The fog lingers. I know I'm out of the hormonal storm, but the emotional debris is everywhere. I feel numb or low or ashamed. I ask myself, "Is this really over? Or is it just hiding around the corner again?" I hesitate to trust the light in me because I know how easily it flickers out. That's the cruel repetition of it. The cycle makes you suspicious of your own joy.

Even in the so-called good days, I sometimes stand in front of the mirror and search. I touch my face like I'm trying to remember how it's supposed to feel. I speak out loud just to hear my own voice and check if it still sounds like me. And some days, it doesn't.

There's a fear that builds inside that silence. A fear that the longer I spend vanishing, the harder it is to come back. That the ghost in the mirror might become permanent. That the real me might eventually give up trying to return at all.

People love to talk about "getting better" as if it's a straight line. They love a tidy redemption arc. But this isn't tidy. This is the same story told again and again, with slight variations. Some chapters are softer. Others are jagged and raw. But the through-line is this question that never fully leaves: Who am I, really, when I keep disappearing?

I wish I had a neat answer. I don't.

All I know is that I keep searching for myself. Even in the hardest weeks, even in the ugliest moments, even when my body is lying and my brain is betraying me, I am still in here somewhere. Still clawing my way back.

Some days, I find her in small rituals. A walk. A song on repeat. Sitting in the same chair by the window where I once wrote something I was proud of. I try not to force it. I try to trust that she'll return when she's ready. I leave the door unlocked.

Other days, I can't feel her at all. And I have to remind myself that being numb doesn't mean I've failed. It just means I'm in the middle of something. It means I'm surviving.

I still see the ghost in the mirror sometimes. But now, I try to soften when I do. I try to say, "Hi. I know it's hard to be here. But we're still here." I try to love the version of me that's lost. Because maybe that's the point. Not to fight so hard to get "back" to something, but to learn how to hold all these versions of myself. Even the haunted ones.

Even the ones that forget who they are.

Because even then, even there, I am still worthy of care. Still worth looking for. And maybe, just maybe, that's what it means to come home.

PART

Two

The Darkness Within

2.1 Rage That Scares Me

Outbursts, Fury, Loss of Control

It doesn't come as a warning. It doesn't tap politely on my shoulder. It crashes through me like a thunderstorm, a roar that turns my blood to fire and makes my own voice foreign to my ears. The rage is not a feeling. It's a possession. A hijacking. Something that turns me into someone I would cross the street to avoid.

One minute I'm ok and the next I'm shaking, shouting, slamming cupboard doors so hard the handles bruise my palms. Someone asks me a simple question and I hear accusation. I hear disrespect. I hear everything I've ever tried to swallow back rise all at once. I bark, I scream, I snap, and I can see the look in their eyes: fear.

Sometimes the rage feels protective. Like it's shielding me from something I haven't even processed yet. But most of the time, it feels shameful. Disproportionate. Wild. I hate it. I hate how it makes me act. I hate how I justify it in the moment, only to crumble with regret an hour later.

It doesn't take much. The wrong tone. A slightly late response. A misplaced item. And suddenly I'm in a different place. A red place. I have yelled so loudly my throat has gone hoarse. I have hurled words like weapons and watched them land. And even while it's happening, even as the storm is breaking, some tiny part of me is aware that this is too much. That I've lost control. That I've handed the wheel to something else.

This isn't ordinary anger. This is something primal. It feels like being cornered with no exit, teeth bared, survival on the line. I feel like I need to defend myself, even when no threat exists. I become defensive over imagined slights, accusatory over neutral words. I turn molehills into mountains and then set them on fire.

It's hardest when it's directed at the people I love. The people who are trying. Who say the wrong thing but mean well. Who don't understand what this is like. Who see only the fury, not the fear beneath it. Afterward I apologize, again and again, but it never feels like enough. Because I know how it felt to them. I know what I looked like. I saw the way they recoiled.

Then comes the shame. The grief. The ache of knowing I scared someone I love. That I damaged something I care about. I try to explain it. "It wasn't me." "I didn't mean it." "It's hormonal." But how do you tell someone you feel possessed and expect them to trust you again? How do you soothe the damage when you don't fully understand it yourself?

This rage isn't just loud. Sometimes it's quiet. Sometimes it seethes under the surface, clenched jaws and bitten tongues, rage turned inward. I slam doors in my head instead of out loud. I fantasize about destruction. I want to disappear so I don't hurt anyone else. I tell myself I'm unlovable. That no one should have to deal with this. That I am a monster wrapped in soft skin.

There have been times I've scared myself. Times I've screamed into pillows until my voice cracked. Times I've hit things just to release the energy. Not people. Never people. But walls, cushions, car steering wheels. Just to feel something break that wasn't me.

PMDD rage is chemical. It's not drama. It's not manipulation. It's not a lack of gratitude or control. It's a physiological hell. A misfiring brain caught in a hormonal noose. And when the switch flips, it's almost impossible to stop the flood. No coping tool, no mantra, no breathing exercise has ever held back a tidal wave. Sometimes I can manage it after the peak, when the worst has passed. But in the middle of it? I am lost.

Yet, even in the middle of it, I still feel the guilt starting to build. I'll be mid-rage and already imagining the apology. Already wondering how to undo what I'm doing. Already hating myself for not being stronger.

There's no victory in surviving these moments. Only survival. I can feel my body buzzing for hours afterward. My heart races like I've run a marathon. My nervous system is raw. And I know it'll come again. The cycle repeats. The storm builds. And no matter how many times I've lived through it, I'm never prepared for how intense it will be.

People say, "You just need to calm down." Or, "You're overreacting." Or, "It's not that serious." But they don't see what's underneath. They don't feel the charge inside my bones. The fire that makes it hard to think clearly. The pulse that beats in my ears louder than reason.

I don't want to be this way. I never chose it. I've spent so much time trying to understand it, trying to outwit it, trying to medicate and meditate and navigate it. But sometimes all I can do is ride it out and pick up the pieces afterward. Apologize. Explain. Cry in the shower. Try again.

This rage is not the whole of me. But in the worst days, it can feel like the only part that matters. The part people remember. The part I can't escape.

If you've felt this, if you've scared yourself, I need you to know you are not evil. You are not broken beyond repair. You are responding to a storm inside your brain. You are doing your best. Even when your best looks like surviving the hour without screaming. Even when your best means walking away mid-argument just to keep the damage minimal.

I am still learning how to forgive myself for what this condition has taken from me. For the damage it's done to my relationships, my confidence, my self-image. But I hold onto the truth that I am not my rage. That I am still worthy of love. Still capable of healing. Still human.

And if this chapter makes you feel seen, even a little, then maybe we are already healing. Together.

2.2 The Weight of the Void
Hopelessness, Emptiness, Suicidal Thoughts

There are days when everything is so quiet. Not the peaceful kind of quiet. Not the silence of calm or rest. This quiet is sterile. Cold. It wraps around me like fog and dulls everything it touches. The colours of the world drain. My thoughts flatten. There is no music in anything.

It doesn't start as a dramatic crash. It creeps in. A slow erosion. I stop replying to messages. I stare at my breakfast until it goes cold. I find myself standing in the middle of the room with no idea what I was supposed to be doing. Nothing feels real. Nothing feels important. I am a ghost in my own life.

This is what the void feels like.

Sometimes it follows the rage, like the comedown after a violent storm. Other times it appears first, a heavy stillness that makes even breathing feel like a task. It's not sadness exactly. Sadness has shape. Sadness wants something. This is different. This is emptiness. It is absence. It is the hollow behind my ribs where my self should be.

I try to explain it and the words fall short. I say, "I'm just tired." Or, "I don't feel like myself today." But what I mean is, I don't feel like anything. I don't know who I am beneath this fog. I can't feel connection. I can't feel joy. Even pain feels muted.

Sometimes I look at the people I love and feel nothing. Not because I don't love them, but because my body won't let me access it. And then the guilt begins. The shame. The fear that I am losing something essential. I wonder if it's permanent. I wonder if this is who I really am underneath it all. I start to believe the lie that I am too broken to function.

The worst part is the way it convinces me I have always felt this way and always will. That this is the truth and everything else was delusion. That the laughter, the connection, the hope I once felt were tricks of the light. PMDD has this way of time-travelling. It rewrites your memories, makes the whole of life feel contaminated.

This is when the thoughts come.

They don't shout. They whisper. You are too much. You are not enough. You are a burden. You ruin everything. You can't keep doing this. The idea of escape begins to seem like mercy. A way to stop hurting people. A way to finally rest.

I have never wanted to die. Not really. What I have wanted is for this pain to end. For the weight of it to lift. For my brain to stop attacking me. I have fantasised about not existing. About dissolving. About stepping out of this body and vanishing into silence. These are not dramatic thoughts. They are slow and convincing. They feel like solutions.

I have sat on the edge of my bed and thought, If I didn't wake up tomorrow, maybe that would be better. And then immediately hated myself for thinking it. I have cried for hours because I know I am loved, and still, the emptiness feels louder. That contradiction is the cruellest part. Being surrounded by good things and still wanting to disappear.

I know I'm not alone in this. I know that others with PMDD carry this same silent weight. I've read their stories. I've seen the pain behind their eyes. Too many of us have had moments when we genuinely believed the world would be better without us. Too many of us have not made it through.

This condition kills. And not just metaphorically. It steals futures. It convinces beautiful, intelligent, loving people that they are nothing. That there is no way out. That there is no point in asking for help because help won't work.

I am still here. Somehow. Even after those thoughts. Even after the days where brushing my teeth felt impossible. Even after weeks where I moved through the world like a shell.

I have clung to the smallest things. The sound of a friend's voice. A song I forgot I loved. The soft warmth of a pet lying beside me. I have written angry poems in the margins of notebooks. I have screamed in the car. I have walked until my feet hurt just to prove to myself I still exist. I have survived, not because I am stronger than anyone else, but because somewhere, some part of me refused to let the void win.

If you have ever felt like this, I want you to hear this part clearly.

You are not a failure if you've had these thoughts. Suicidal ideation is a symptom. It is not a truth. It is not a prediction. It is not who you are.

PMDD distorts perception. It magnifies fear. It mutes joy. It isolates. And in that isolation, it breeds hopelessness. But that hopelessness is not permanent. You can come back from it. I have. More than once. And I will again.

The key is remembering that these thoughts, as convincing as they feel, are not facts. They are a product of a brain in survival mode. A body caught in a hormonal undertow. And help is possible. Not just platitudes. Real, gritty, compassionate help. Through therapy. Through medication. Through connection. Through talking to someone who understands.

When the void comes, I try to treat myself like I would a friend. I don't always succeed. But I try. I remind myself that this feeling has passed before. That it is part of a cycle, not a sentence. I make plans with my future self. I write letters to the version of me who will feel joy again. Because I always do. Even if I forget it in the dark.

If you're in the middle of it now, hold on. Hold on with both hands. Tell someone. Whisper it if you have to. You don't need to be strong. You just need to stay. The world needs you. Not just the version of you who smiles. The whole of you. Even this version. Especially this version.

Because you are not the void. You are the one surviving it.

2.3 Crisis Mode

What to Do When You're at the Edge

I always know when it starts.

The thoughts stop asking and start demanding. When your body is frozen or frantic, your chest tight, your mind loud and fast or terrifyingly blank. This is the edge. The cliff. The moment when everything feels too much, and you start to wonder if you can survive even one more hour like this.

If you are there now, stop reading for insight and start reading for survival. I am not here to offer platitudes. I am not here to hand you pretty words that don't stick. I am here to sit with you in it. To speak to you as someone who has stood on that same edge, shaking, and lived.

First, you need to remember that thoughts are not actions. They can scream, they can ache, they can beg you to listen, but they are still only thoughts. They are symptoms. They are not prophecies. You are allowed to have them and still choose to stay. You are allowed to feel like you want to disappear and still find a reason to take another breath.

So, what do you do in crisis mode? When the pain is louder than reason? When every part of you is screaming to shut it down?

You ground.

Not perfectly. Not magically. Just enough to interrupt the spiral. Start with what's real around you. Look around the room. Name five things you can see. A chair. A cup. A crack in the wall. A piece of lint. Anything. Then four things you can feel. Your feet on the floor. Your shirt against your skin. The burn behind your eyes. The cool air on your hands. Then listen. Name three sounds. Your breath. The hum of the fridge. Distant traffic. Then smell. Then taste. Doesn't matter if it feels stupid. Doesn't matter if you don't believe it will help. Just do it.

You are not fixing yourself in this moment. You are anchoring. You are choosing to stay for one more minute. And then the next.

If that doesn't work, or even if it does, try movement. Any movement. Punch a pillow. Sit on the floor and press your back against the wall. Put your hands in cold water. Walk around the room ten times. Shake your arms out. Jump. Dance with rage. Movement interrupts the feedback loop of panic. It reminds the body that it is still alive.

Now tell someone. If that feels too big, send a one-word message. "Help." "Crisis." "Here." Choose someone you trust. Or call a helpline. You do not need to explain everything. You do not need to justify your pain. You just need to say, "I'm not okay." The act of reaching out is enough.

There is no shame in crisis. None. You are not weak for getting here. You are not broken. You are experiencing a state of emergency inside your body. You deserve the same care and urgency as anyone else in pain. If you had a heart attack, you wouldn't try to walk it off. Don't try to "handle" this alone.

Write down what helps, so you don't have to think later. Make a crisis plan for yourself. Stick it to your mirror. Save it in your phone. Include names of people you trust. Include helpline numbers. Include reminders like: "You have felt this way before, and it passed." "This is a medical state, not a personal failure." "You are needed. You are loved. You are not a burden." Even if you don't believe it right now, write it anyway. Future you will need it.

If you can, get outside. Feel the ground. Stare at a tree, a leaf, the cracks in the pavement. Anything that reminds you the world is still turning. If you can't get outside, open a window. Let in air. Let in light. Sit where you can see the sky.

If you're alone and scared, make a pact with yourself. One hour. Just stay one more hour. Then one more. Break it down. Crisis mode is not about fixing your life. It's about surviving the next breath. The next five minutes. That is enough.

It's okay if your brain is saying cruel things right now. You don't have to argue with it. You don't have to believe it either. Just label it. "That's a crisis thought." Let it pass through without giving it weight. You are not what your brain says when it's at war with itself.

And when the wave begins to pass, because it will, even if it doesn't feel like it now, you may feel numb. Exhausted. Raw. That is normal.

Let yourself land softly. Don't rush into fixing everything. Don't punish yourself for the moment you just survived. Drink water. Eat something gentle. Rest. Wrap yourself in something warm. You just made it through a hurricane.

Later, you may feel embarrassed. You may want to hide. But I want you to understand this: what you just went through was not weakness. It was not shameful. It was survival. And that matters. That is sacred. You stayed.

Now is the time to begin thinking about support. Not just when you're in crisis, but before it. You deserve care between the storms, not just during them. That might mean talking to a doctor, trying new treatment, finding a therapist who understands PMDD. It might mean building a circle of people who know the signs and are willing to hold you when it gets too loud.

Crisis mode is terrifying. But it is not the end. I've been there, more than once, and I am still here. There are women reading this right now who have been where you are. We are out here, waiting for you, holding space for your return. You are not alone.

Please stay. The world may not feel like it right now, but it needs your voice. Your laughter. Your weird stories. Your tears. Your truth. You are not done.

Let this chapter be your emergency flare. Let it remind you that someone, somewhere, knows how it feels to be at the edge. And still believes you can make it back. You are still here. That is everything.

PART

Three

The Split Self

3.1 Two Lives, One Body

Follicular vs. Luteal: the Jekyll & Hyde Cycle

There's a sharp kind of ache in living as two people stitched into one skin. The turning point always feels like a crash. It's not a metaphor, or a poetic way of describing a bad mood. It is a physiological, psychological, chemical transformation that happens like clockwork, every month. One week I am calm, focused, full of life. The next, I am pacing, withdrawn, hypersensitive, overwhelmed. Two versions of me, tethered to the same frame. I don't get to choose which one shows up.

In the medical world, it's mapped out in neat diagrams and tidy graphs. The follicular phase, rising estrogen, the brain in relative harmony. Then ovulation. Then the luteal phase, progesterone rising, then crashing, and with it comes the chaos. The truth is more jagged. It doesn't always wait politely for ovulation to finish before the descent begins. It doesn't announce its arrival. One morning I wake up and everything feels just slightly off. And then a landslide.

This cycle is like living with Dr. Jekyll and Mr. Hyde. Except I am both. I am the scientist and the monster. The woman who makes dinner and calls her friends, and the woman who can't answer a single message without trembling. The woman who smiles at strangers and thinks about the future with hope, and the woman who cannot bear to be looked at, who thinks about disappearing. I used to think these moods came from something I did wrong. Maybe I was weak. But

I've learned this is biology, not failure. Still, the knowledge doesn't soften the impact.

The follicular self is the version of me I wish I could always be. She is generous with her time, she laughs with her whole body, she gets things done. She says yes to invitations. She remembers to eat and hydrate. She cares about what she wears and feels things like ambition and curiosity. I see her in the mirror and think, "There you are. You're back." I am suspicious of her now. I've been burned too many times by how fleeting she is. Still, I miss her when she's gone. She is the version people compliment. The version who can go to the shops without sunglasses and earbuds.

The luteal self is something else entirely. Her skin hurts. Her thoughts spiral. She can't trust her perceptions, because everything feels threatening or too loud or deeply, deeply wrong. She pulls back from everything and everyone. She does not feel like herself, but she *is* me. That's the hardest part. The rage doesn't feel justified, but it is real. The despair doesn't have a neat origin, but it consumes everything in its path. Even the smallest thing, spilling tea, forgetting to reply to an email, can send her into meltdown or paralysis.

I've learned to track these changes now. I keep a calendar. I circle the days I know will be dangerous. I try not to schedule anything too demanding around them. I prepare food in advance, write kind notes to myself, cancel plans where I can. It feels a little like living with a chronic invader. One I can't evict, only accommodate.

There are times in the follicular phase when I look back at the luteal days and feel horrified. What did I say? Who did I push away? Why did I think those things about myself? I review the damage and feel shame, even when I know it wasn't entirely under my control. It's like waking up after a storm and finding debris everywhere. I become the clean-up crew for a version of me who didn't mean to destroy anything but did anyway.

And then the cycle repeats.

People think of hormones as background noise, something minor. But in PMDD, they are the main character. They dictate how I experience the world, how I move through it, how I relate to others and to myself. It's not a mood swing. It's a full-body shift. The entire landscape of my mind and body changes. Sensations that were neutral before become painful. Sounds are sharper. My skin is too sensitive. Food tastes off. My sleep is fractured. Everything is a little bit wrong.

This is the Jekyll and Hyde experience of PMDD: one half of the month you're thriving, the other half you're surviving. And the cruelty is in how vividly you *remember* your better self. You don't forget her. You can picture her clearly, which makes the contrast unbearable. In the depths of the luteal phase, you mourn her. You wonder if she's ever coming back. You worry that maybe this time, the darkness is permanent.

I sometimes try to explain this to people, and they look at me like I'm exaggerating. "That's just hormones," they say. Or, "Have you tried meditation?" I wish it were that simple. I have meditated until my body shook with effort. I have taken vitamins, changed my diet, exercised, slept, journaled, fasted, sobbed. I have whispered apologies to the people who love me, because they don't know which version of me they're going to get. Sometimes I don't either.

The follicular self watches the luteal self with sorrow. She wants to help. She wants to believe things won't get that bad again. She wants to forget. But forgetting means being caught off guard again. And so I've stopped pretending I don't know what's coming. I've started treating the cycle with a strange kind of reverence. It's a brutal rhythm, but it's mine. I am learning not to hate the darker self. She is wounded, not wicked. She is carrying pain I don't fully understand. She needs compassion, not correction.

There is no perfect way to reconcile the two. But I am trying. I am trying to build a life that makes space for both versions of me, even if only one of them feels manageable. I am learning that strength isn't pretending everything is fine. It's acknowledging the split and surviving it anyway.

I live two lives. I am one body. I do not have to be whole to be worthy.

"Some women bloom all month. I am a tide, rising, retreating, wrecking, healing. Both are nature. Both are real."

The Strange Calm

The Eerie Return to Normality After the Storm

It never fades. It vanishes.

No warning, no grand reveal, just the sudden lightness of coming back. One morning, I open my eyes and the fog is simply gone. My limbs feel lighter. The air no longer tastes like threat. My brain begins to hum instead of scream. I do not trust it at first.

After days, or sometimes weeks, of chaos, there is something almost unnatural about the quiet that follows. It is not a celebration. It feels like waking up in the aftermath of a disaster, where everything is strangely still and the birds have returned but the wreckage remains. There is no applause for surviving. Just silence.

The strange calm. That is what I have come to call it. It is the period when my body and mind realign. When the floodwaters recede and the debris is left behind. In these first few days of the follicular phase, I don't feel like myself exactly. I feel like someone emerging from captivity, blinking into the sun, unsure whether to hope or brace. The storm is over, but the memory of it clings.

It's bizarre how normal things suddenly become possible again. I can make a phone call. I can laugh at a joke. I can answer an email without crying. I can feel hunger, make breakfast, brush my hair. I can plan the day without dreading it. But every action is watched by a part of me that remembers the person I was just a few days before. That shadow still lingers at the edge of the mirror.

The body is so convincing in its recovery. The skin feels less raw. My heart stops racing at shadows. The rage that once flared like wildfire now feels absurd. I look back on the things I said, the thoughts I had, the tears I shed over tiny triggers, and I feel shame. Embarrassment. Even disbelief. Was that really me? Did I really fall apart that hard, again?

This is part of the cruelty. The return to normality comes with a haunting. I don't just get relief, I get the burden of remembering what I became. What I felt. What I did or didn't say. Who I pushed away. And I am always terrified that they noticed. That someone saw through the excuses, the cancelled plans, the silence. That someone is keeping score.

The strange calm is full of questions. How bad was it this time? Did I damage anything I care about? Is there something I need to fix, to explain, to undo? But also: how long do I have before it happens again? That is the quiet dread pulsing beneath the peace. How many good days do I get before I lose myself again?

It would be easier if I could pretend it was all over. That this is the new baseline and the storm will never return. But I have been through too many cycles to believe that lie. So I begin the slow work of patching things together again. I reply to messages I ignored. I resurface in conversations. I wash clothes. I look at the to-do list with new energy and try not to feel overwhelmed by what was missed.

There is also guilt in this phase. The guilt of having to re-enter the world and pretend everything is fine. The guilt of looking healthy when I was not, just days ago. The guilt of functioning again when I know people around me may not have seen the full picture. I want to shout, "You have no idea what I just survived." But I don't. I carry it quietly. Most of us do.

This in-between space, this eerie calm, is oddly fragile. I want to lean into it, to enjoy the return of peace, but I also feel like I'm walking on thin ice. There's a cautiousness to it. Like I might wake up tomorrow and find that it was a trick. That I misread the signals. That I am not better, only momentarily reprieved. So I move slowly. I listen to my body with suspicion. I hope with restraint.

Sometimes, I feel almost euphoric in this phase. Not in a manic way, but in the kind of gentle high that comes from having your own mind returned to you. There is a clarity I haven't felt in weeks. Thoughts that once swirled like a blizzard now land softly. Ideas come back. Dreams return. I feel inspired, even joyful. It's like the world is vivid again, as if someone adjusted the brightness. I want to capture it. Bottle it. Save it for when the next darkness arrives.

But I also know this phase is where people forget. Not just others, but me too. The pain recedes and I start to question how bad it really was. Maybe I exaggerated it. Maybe I was just tired. Maybe it's gone for good. Maybe it wasn't that serious. This is dangerous. Because forgetting means I won't be prepared. Forgetting means I'll blame myself again next time. So I write things down. I keep records. I remind myself of the reality.

The strange calm teaches me a lot. It reminds me that I am not only the storm. That there is a version of me who is steady and thoughtful and kind. That the darkness doesn't erase her, even if it drowns her voice for a while. It also teaches me how resilient I am. Not in a shiny, Instagram-worthy way. In a quiet, relentless way. The kind of strength that no one sees, because it happens behind closed doors. In silence. In survival.

I am learning to honour the strange calm. To not fill it immediately with tasks and guilt and fixing. I am learning to rest here. To let myself feel the relief. To trust that this peace, however fleeting, is real while it lasts. I do not have to earn it. I do not have to apologise for it. I can just be.

This return to normality is not the end of the story. It is the intermission. A breath between waves. A soft, tentative truce between biology and self. I will take it.

Even if it is strange.
Even if it is short.

3.3 Who Am I the Rest of the Time?
Rebuilding Identity Between Episodes

It's a strange question to ask yourself in adulthood: *Who am I, really?*

Not in the abstract sense, but in a practical, aching way. Who am I when I'm not crying into my pillow or losing my temper at something harmless? Who am I when I'm not pacing the room, checking my pulse, convinced I'm falling apart? Who is the version of me that exists between the collapses?

Living with PMDD fractures your identity. Not in a poetic, soul-searching way, but in a real, unsettling sense. You spend half your month surviving, and the other half trying to piece together what's left of you. Somewhere in between the hormonal violence and the short-lived peace, there's a sliver of time. A stretch of days that feels neutral. Not quite joyful, not quite dark. Just… quiet. It is there that I find myself asking: is this who I really am?

Because the truth is, I don't always know. My memories of myself are blurred by mood. When I feel good, I remember myself as hopeful, kind, curious. When I feel awful, I remember being difficult, sharp, unbearable. The cycle colours my self-perception so deeply that it's hard to find a version of me that feels consistent. Some days, I wonder if there *is* a real me at all, or just phases pretending to be people.

During those more stable stretches, days without tears, without panic, without fury, I catch glimpses. I remember what I like. What I'm drawn to. I read books that stir something in me. I laugh, not performatively but with my whole chest. I go for walks and feel connected to the sky again. I notice colours. I remember the names of people I love. And I think: maybe this is it. Maybe this is who I am.

The identity never stays fixed. Just as I start to find a rhythm, the ground shifts beneath me. I am reminded that everything I rebuild might be swept away again. So, I start small. I try not to build palaces out of passing moods. I learn to anchor myself in what stays true. I am someone who loves dogs. I feel better near water. I find comfort in notebooks and soft clothes and afternoon light. These are facts I can return to, even when I cannot return to myself.

Rebuilding identity while living through PMDD is like patching a house that floods every month. You keep trying to make it liveable, even knowing the next storm will come. You put up photographs, plant herbs on the windowsill, hang wind chimes. You make it yours anyway. Because if you wait for permanent safety, you may never start living.

There is also grief in this. I grieve the stability that others seem to take for granted. The ability to be one version of themselves all the time. I wonder what kind of career I'd have had by now. What kind of partner I'd be. What I could have created with all those stolen days. But grief is not the same as failure. Feeling the loss does not mean I have nothing left. In fact, it means I cared. It means I still care.

Sometimes I talk to friends about identity. About how we form ourselves through the roles we play: worker, lover, parent, artist, friend. But when your condition steals those roles from you temporarily, when you cannot show up, cannot create, cannot speak kindly, cannot cope, it shakes the foundation. I wonder if people still see me the same. I wonder if I am still *me* if I am not doing the things that make me feel like myself.

That's why I've learned to define myself more gently. Not by how productive I am, or how consistent I can be, but by how I return. By how I keep coming back to myself, again and again, even when I've been pulled away by the current. I am the person who returns. I am the person who tries. That counts for something.

And on the days when I feel most lost, I ask smaller questions. Not *who am I?* but *what soothes me? What helps? What do I long for right now?* These are easier to answer. They bring me back into the room. Sometimes the answer is tea. Or a familiar film. Or sunlight. Or letting myself cry without shame. In those tiny answers, identity begins to grow again.

There is power in refusing to let PMDD be the full definition of me. Yes, it is a massive force in my life. Yes, it dictates how I feel for a significant portion of every month. But it is not everything. I am not just the woman who breaks. I am the woman who writes about it.

Who reaches for meaning. Who sees beauty, even after the storm. Who dares to laugh again, even if it won't last.

Rebuilding identity is not a single act. It is a practice. I learn who I am through repetition. Through patterns. Through moments when I surprise myself. Through the softening I feel when I look at old photos and remember I have always been trying. Through the music that still moves me. Through the friendships that hold me even when I go silent for days. Through the words I write when I cannot speak out loud.

And yes, some days I feel like a stranger to myself. But even strangers can become familiar. I am learning to meet myself with curiosity instead of dread. To ask, *What version of me is here today?* and then move from there. I do not always like the answer, but I do try to listen.

There is a self beneath the suffering. Not separate from it, but deeper. A self who holds the memory of who I was before it all got complicated. A self who dreams of a future where the waves are softer, where the cycle is gentler. She is still here, even when the rest of me is unravelling.

And so, between episodes, I build. With softness. With slowness. With grace. I build a version of me that is not perfect, but real. Not unshakable, but willing. I build a self who can hold both the darkness and the light, and who does not vanish completely when the storm comes.

I may never have the stability I once imagined. But I have something else. I have the strength to begin again. Every month. Every time.

That, too, is identity.

PART

Four

---⟩ ○ ⟨---

Gaslighted by Biology

4.1 "It's Just Hormones"
The Dangerous Minimising of PMDD

Don't say it's just hormones, you don't understand.
This storm isn't mild, it's swallowing land.
It tears through the calm with a venomous scream,
Stealing my mind and infecting my dreams.

Don't call me too sensitive, fragile, or weak.
You didn't see me lose days I can't speak.
You weren't there when I shook in my bed,
Scared of the thoughts that screamed in my head.

Don't tell me to breathe or to just let it slide.
You can't fight a war that's raging inside.
I need truth, not dismissal dressed up as care,
Call it by name, or don't even dare.

"Don't tell me I'm overreacting while I'm surviving a biochemical betrayal."

There are few phrases more infuriating to someone with PMDD than this one: *It's just hormones.* Three small words. Soft on the surface. Insidious underneath. This phrase has been weaponised for generations to silence, belittle, and discredit people experiencing extreme hormonal suffering. It's whispered in clinics. Scoffed across kitchen tables. Laughed off in workplaces. Shrugged away in emergency rooms. And every time it's spoken, it erases the true devastation of PMDD and replaces it with a lie: that we are simply too sensitive, too emotional, too weak to handle something supposedly natural.

Let us be clear. PMDD is not *just* hormones. It is a hormone-based *disorder*. A neuroendocrine condition. A premenstrual death spiral. It is not a mild inconvenience or a quirky personality shift. PMDD is a life-altering condition that can dismantle your career, sabotage your relationships, and leave you sobbing on a bathroom floor wondering if you'll make it to morning. It deserves seriousness. It deserves compassion. It deserves recognition.

Yet time and again, it is trivialised. Minimized into cliché. Wrapped up in a bow of tired stereotypes about moody women, raging wives, and chocolate cravings. You try to explain your symptoms, the despair, the dissociation, the volcanic rage, the suicidal thoughts, and what you get in return is a smirk and a dismissal: "Ah, hormones. We've all been there." As if you're not bleeding out inside your own mind. As if you haven't thought about ending your life three times this week. As if your brain hasn't turned into a war zone where you no longer know who you are.

The danger of this minimising isn't just emotional. It's systemic. When something is dismissed as *just hormones*, it doesn't get researched. It doesn't get funded. It doesn't get taken seriously in medical training. Doctors don't learn about it properly. Mental health professionals overlook it. GPs confuse it with PMS or anxiety. And people with PMDD are left undiagnosed, untreated, and gaslit, sometimes for decades. There are still individuals in their thirties and forties discovering this diagnosis for the first time, after years of thinking they were broken beyond repair.

The system is broken.

Too many of us have internalised the message that we are exaggerating. That we are making it up. That we are the problem. So, we learn to mask. To downplay. To swallow our pain and smile through it. We don't cry for help until we're in absolute crisis, and by then, the damage has been done. Some of us don't make it out.

This is why the phrase "It's just hormones" is not just ignorant. It is dangerous. It delays diagnosis. It prevents treatment. It isolates sufferers. It fosters shame. And worst of all, it tells people that their suffering doesn't count. That their pain is normal and should be endured quietly. That they are hysterical, unbalanced, or weak.

But those of us living with PMDD are none of those things. We are fighters. We are survivors. We are navigating a condition that hijacks our brains and tries to kill us every month, and still, we show up. Still, we care for others. Still, we try to hold our lives together even as they fall apart like clockwork. That is strength. That is resilience. And it deserves to be seen.

Let's talk about the real impact of PMDD. Not the diluted version. The real thing.

It's missing days of work because you're too mentally unstable to function, but too ashamed to say why.

It's snapping at someone you love and watching the confusion in their eyes while a part of you screams internally: *This isn't me. Please believe me.*

It's waking up with a leaden weight in your chest, unsure why you feel so broken, until you check your calendar and realise: it's that time again.

It's holding a prescription in one hand and a crisis plan in the other, wondering which one will save you this time.

None of that is *just* anything.

Hormones are powerful. They are not minor players in the human body. They are chemical messengers that affect every system, brain, mood, digestion, sleep, pain, memory, and beyond. In PMDD, the brain is unusually sensitive to the normal fluctuations of progesterone and estrogen. This sensitivity sets off a cascade of neurological chaos. Mood-regulating chemicals misfire. The limbic system flares. Cognitive distortion sets in. Suicidal ideation is not uncommon. And it all happens with horrifying predictability.

This isn't a character flaw. This isn't an attitude problem. This isn't something a hot bath and a yoga class can fix.

This is a medical condition. A serious one.

And yet, people with PMDD still find themselves begging to be heard. Being told to "relax," to "toughen up," to "stop being so dramatic." Would someone with epilepsy be spoken to this way? Or someone with diabetes? Would we tell someone in the middle of a seizure to breathe through it and think positive? Of course not. But because PMDD is hormonal, and hormonal has been feminised, and feminised has been devalued, it becomes invisible.

We're here to shine a light on it.

We're here to reject the narrative that our bodies are betraying us because we are weak.

We're here to say that hormone-based disorders deserve research, respect, and radical change in the way we talk about women's health.

No more minimising.

No more brushing it off.

No more normalising monthly collapse.

It's not *just hormones* when your mental health plummets every few weeks.

It's not *just hormones* when your personality fractures and you become unrecognisable to yourself.

It's not *just hormones* when your life begins to revolve around surviving the next episode.

And it's not *just hormones* when the thing inside your body that's supposed to sustain life instead threatens it.

It's PMDD. It's real. It's serious. And it deserves to be named, understood, and treated with the full force of medicine, compassion, and truth.

If anyone ever tells you it's *just hormones*, look them straight in the eye and say: No, it's not. It's hell. And I'm still here.

That is nothing short of heroic.

4.2 Misdiagnosed, Mistreated

Depression, BPD, Bipolar... but Never Quite Right

There is an utter madness that comes from knowing something is deeply wrong inside you and having the world mislabel it, over and over again.

For many of us with PMDD, the journey to diagnosis is not a straight line. It's a maze. Twisting corridors of guesswork, assumptions, and shrugged shoulders. We arrive in doctor's offices carrying the weight of our pain and confusion, desperate for clarity, only to leave with a prescription and a new label that never quite fits.

Depression.

Anxiety.

Borderline Personality Disorder.

Bipolar Disorder.

We collect these diagnoses like scars. Some of them stay with us for years. Some become cages. Others get discarded after months of trying to explain, once again, that this version of ourselves only exists for part of the month. That the darkness isn't constant. That the emptiness comes in waves. That there is a pattern to the chaos, if only someone would listen long enough to see it.

Most professionals are trained to see symptoms, not cycles. They hear about suicidal thoughts and reach for the DSM. They don't ask about periods. They don't track dates. They don't connect the dots between hormones and mental health. So instead of being seen in full, we are fragmented.

When you say you feel okay half the time but like a completely different person the rest, you sound like someone with mood instability. When you describe intense emotional reactions, overwhelming sensitivity, fear of abandonment, or rage that scares you, some therapists reach for the BPD stamp without digging any deeper.

If you've ever heard the phrase *You seem to fit the criteria* but felt in your bones that it wasn't the whole story, you are not alone.

The misdiagnosis of PMDD is not rare. It is epidemic.

Because PMDD mimics many other conditions, depression, anxiety disorders, bipolar II, complex PTSD, it often gets lost in the noise. And because many of us don't even know PMDD exists, we don't know what to ask for. We walk into clinics thinking maybe we *are* mentally ill, maybe permanently. We doubt ourselves. We believe the labels. We try the treatments.

Antidepressants that dull us to the world.

Mood stabilisers that numb without lifting.

Therapy modalities that never quite land because they are treating a symptom, not a cycle.

We learn to live around the misdiagnosis. We build coping strategies that aren't tailored to our condition. We accept half-healing because that's all we've ever been offered. We sit in support groups and wonder why our stories don't match the others. We swallow medications that bring little relief and side effects that feel like new problems stacked on top of old ones.

And when things don't improve, the problem gets pinned on us.

You're resistant to treatment.

You're non-compliant.

You're not trying hard enough.

The sad truth is, we've been trying for years. Sometimes decades. We've journaled. We've meditated. We've done trauma work. We've gone on and off medications. We've tried clean eating, exercise, CBT, prayer, fasting, supplements, abstinence. We have tried everything under the sun, except the one thing that actually explains why our suffering has a schedule.

Because no one thought to ask about hormones.

This silence around PMDD is a form of medical negligence. When a condition affects one in twenty people with ovaries and still goes unrecognised by the majority of healthcare professionals, something is broken.

Some of us discover PMDD through a chance article, a TikTok, a throwaway comment on a forum. A mirror suddenly held up to us by accident. We look into it and feel the shock of recognition. The lightbulb moment. The timelines line up. The two-week crash makes sense. The erratic mood shifts have a rhythm now. For the first time, we are not confused.

The relief is short-lived, because validation is not the same as support.

You take this discovery to your doctor, and they look blank. They've barely heard of it. Maybe they say it's not real. Maybe they confuse it with PMS. Maybe they offer you antidepressants again, or the Pill, or tell you to "wait and see."

Or worse, they laugh it off.

We all get a bit hormonal.

The lack of understanding is enraging. It is disempowering. It makes you feel invisible.

But you are not.

You are here.

You are part of a community of people who have been gaslit by medicine and forced to become their own experts. You are not imagining things. You are not exaggerating. If your diagnosis has never quite fit, if the treatments have never quite worked, if your symptoms seem to rise and fall like tides, that is not a coincidence.

It is a cycle.

And cycles demand a different kind of care.

True PMDD treatment begins with recognition. Not just of the condition, but of the harm done by misdiagnosis. There is grief in realising how many years were lost to the wrong lens. There is rage, too. Rightfully so. Because we should have been seen. We should have been believed. We should not have had to suffer through identities that weren't ours, through medications that didn't help, through labels that added stigma to our pain.

You are allowed to be angry. You are allowed to be heartbroken. You are allowed to reclaim your story.

PMDD is real. And it is not the same as depression, even though it can feel just as dark. It is not BPD, though it can shake your sense of self. It is not bipolar, although it can swing you between highs and lows. PMDD has its own signature. Its own rhythm. Its own havoc.

It deserves its own name.

The more we speak up, the harder it becomes for the medical world to ignore us. The more accurate our diagnoses become, the more precise our treatments can be. And the more people we can save, not just from the condition, but from the years of confusion and despair that come with being told you are something you are not.

If this is your story, you are not alone. You are not broken. You were never misbehaving. You were misdiagnosed.

And now, you get to write a new chapter. One where the name is right. One where you are finally seen.

4.3 The Fight for Belief

Standing Up to Be Taken Seriously

There comes a moment in nearly every PMDD journey when silence becomes unbearable. When you've swallowed your pain for too long. When you've smiled through symptoms that have tried to destroy you. When you're done being dismissed, ignored, or told it's all in your head. That moment is the beginning of the fight for belief.

And make no mistake, it is a fight.

To have PMDD is to know the burden of proof is constantly placed on your shoulders. You must explain, defend, track, document, advocate, and re-explain your own suffering. Again and again. To doctors, to employers, to family, to friends, to partners. Sometimes even to yourself.

Because the world does not take hormonal disorders seriously.

Because pain that fluctuates is considered suspect.

Because if you look fine some of the time, people assume you're exaggerating the rest of the time.

And because you have ovaries, your distress is automatically downgraded. Reframed as drama. Labelled as emotional. Treated as temporary. This is the legacy of a system that still sees female-bodied health issues as secondary. Optional. Too complicated to bother with.

But PMDD is not optional. It is not a "women's issue." It is a full-body, full-brain disorder that can unravel your life on a reliable schedule. And it deserves the same seriousness as any other condition that threatens your wellbeing, your career, your relationships, and your will to live.

So we speak up. Sometimes for the first time. Sometimes through tears. Sometimes with shaking voices. Sometimes with all the rage we've carried in our bodies for years.

We say: I am not okay. And I need you to believe me.

And often, the world says: Are you sure? Isn't it just PMS? Maybe you're overreacting. Maybe you're stressed. Maybe you should try yoga. Maybe you should calm down.

As if calming down is a cure for biochemical chaos.

This is where so many of us hit the wall. We come forward, only to be doubted. We bring receipts, symptom trackers, cycle maps, mood charts, only to be met with vague reassurance or blank confusion. We are sent home with antidepressants, or told to go on the Pill, or worse, told that nothing can be done.

It is enraging.

It is exhausting.

And it is the precise reason why people with PMDD have had to become warriors.

We've had to educate ourselves more thoroughly than some of the doctors we see. We've had to memorise medical research, understand hormone interactions, read clinical guidelines, and become fluent in the language of psychiatry and gynaecology just to get a foothold in a system that should have caught us years ago.

We've had to print studies and bring them to appointments like weapons.

We've had to track our symptoms for months just to get someone to listen.

We've had to advocate for ourselves when we were at our lowest, barely functioning, on the edge of survival.

And even then, we are told we are too much. Too angry. Too intense. Too dramatic.

But here's the truth they don't want to say out loud: anger is appropriate. When your suffering is minimised. When your life is shaped by an undiagnosed condition. When you're drowning and everyone around you is telling you it's just a puddle. Of course you're angry. That anger is fuel. That anger is sacred. That anger is a compass pointing directly to injustice.

You have every right to demand to be taken seriously.

Your pain is real.

Your symptoms are not up for debate.

Your experience matters, even if it doesn't fit the convenient narrative.

The fight for belief is about reclaiming your story. It is about standing in front of a world that repeatedly tries to silence you and saying, No. I won't be quiet. I won't pretend this is fine. I won't sit down while my condition is brushed aside because it's messy, complicated, or hormonal.

You deserve more than platitudes. You deserve research. You deserve treatment options. You deserve to be believed the first time you say, "Something is wrong."

But belief often comes second, after battle. And that battle can be long. It might look like changing doctors until one finally understands. It might mean losing relationships with people who never tried to understand. It might mean confronting bosses who mock your sick days, or friends who vanish when you are not your best self.

Standing up for yourself does not always bring applause. But it does bring freedom.

The moment you stop shrinking your truth to fit other people's comfort, things begin to change. You step into your power. You begin to connect with others who know the storm. You stop internalising the gaslighting. You stop apologising for surviving.

And most importantly, you begin to trust yourself again.

Because belief starts inside. That is the core of this fight. When the world has told you over and over that you are exaggerating, overreacting, or imagining things, it takes fierce courage to stand up and say: I believe myself. I believe my body. I believe my experience.

That belief is radical. That belief is power.

So if you are in the middle of the fight, still seeking diagnosis, still pushing for care, still demanding recognition, know this:

There is a whole army of us standing with you. We see you. We believe you. We've been where you are.

And if you are on the other side of that fight, never stop speaking your truth. Your voice is a lighthouse for someone still in the dark.

We live in a world where hormonal suffering is still hidden, still mocked, still erased. But we are changing that. With every story shared. With every no more. With every brave, exhausted person who refuses to stay silent.

This is the fight for belief.

And we are winning.

PART

Five

---))　○　((---

Collateral Damage

5.1 Broken Relationships

When the people you love don't understand

It's a different kind of heartbreak, not from being abandoned, but from being seen as someone you're not.

Someone scary.
Someone fragile.

Someone they no longer recognise.

PMDD doesn't just take a toll on your mind. It stretches its fingers into the fabric of your closest relationships and starts pulling at the seams. It distorts your words, heightens your reactions, exhausts your ability to communicate gently. And when the people you love most don't understand that, the result is often one you never meant: distance, confusion, silence.

There are things I've said that I can't take back. There are messages I didn't send because I didn't trust myself to be kind. There are people who meant the world to me, and now they are gone. Not because I didn't love them, but because love alone couldn't withstand the storm.

Sometimes they leave because they think you're toxic. Sometimes they stay just long enough to let you know you've changed, and not in a good way. They say things like "you're so dramatic lately," or "I never know which version of you I'm going to get." And they mean it as a complaint, not a cry for help.

The truth is, you don't know which version of you they're going to get either.

You try to explain. You tell them it's hormonal. You tell them you're not choosing this. You even show them the calendar, point to the dates, circle them in red, and say, "See? This is when it happens. It always happens. Can't you see it's not me?"

But they don't see. They just see the words you screamed, the tears you couldn't explain, the way you shut down for days or lashed out without warning. They see your withdrawal as punishment. They see your volatility as a flaw in your character. They don't see the war happening inside you.

Some friendships disappear slowly. A message goes unanswered. A phone call doesn't come. Invitations stop. You're no longer someone they feel safe with. Or maybe you were always the one chasing, and now you've stopped running after people who wouldn't look back.

Romantic relationships? Those are a different battlefield entirely. Loving someone with PMDD requires deep, unwavering patience. It means being okay with the fact that you will be blamed, sometimes unfairly, by someone who feels like they are drowning. It means weathering the storm without making it about yourself. And most people simply don't have that kind of stamina.

You see them flinch when you raise your voice. You see their disappointment when you cancel plans. You see the light in their eyes dim when you try to explain again what you're going through and they say, "But you were fine yesterday."

You know they love you. But love alone doesn't mean they'll stay. And sometimes, you don't blame them for leaving. Not really. You know what it feels like to live inside your body during those weeks. It's hell. Why would anyone else choose to step into the fire with you?

And still, it hurts. Deeply. It feels like being abandoned for something you can't control. Like being punished for an illness. Like being told your suffering is too loud, too inconvenient, too uncomfortable to witness.

Sometimes the guilt is heavier than the rage. You replay the moment you snapped, even though you were trying to be calm. You remember the look on their face. You see the text you wrote in fury and wish you had deleted it. You think, *maybe I am too much. Maybe I don't deserve closeness.*

But that isn't the truth. The truth is, PMDD creates a wound that reopens every month. And when you are bleeding out, it is hard to love anyone properly. It's hard to be soft. It's hard to be reasonable. You are surviving. And survival rarely looks gentle.

Some people are never going to understand that. They will label you as unstable. They will distance themselves for their own protection.

And while that might be their right, it still carves out an ache in you. An ache that doesn't heal easily.

Other times, people want to help, but they do it badly. They say things like "Just try to be more positive," or "You need to control your emotions." They love you, but they don't take the time to learn. They think your sadness is something you can snap out of. They think your rage is a choice. And slowly, you stop confiding in them. You stop trusting them to hold your pain. The space between you grows.

There are relationships I still grieve. Friendships that were once filled with laughter but couldn't survive the silence that PMDD brought. Family members who watched me suffer but never asked how they could support me. Partners who loved the bright version of me and couldn't face the one that came after ovulation.

The hardest part is feeling like *you* were the one who ruined it. Like your body's betrayal became your personal failing. And in that shame, you isolate further. You begin to believe you are safer alone. That maybe love is not something you can afford while battling this.

But here's what I've learned, painfully and slowly: the people who are meant to stay will stay. Not without struggle. Not without mistakes. But they will try. They will listen. They will research. They will ask questions. They will apologise when they get it wrong. And most importantly, they won't weaponize your symptoms against you.

They won't make your pain your identity.

They won't walk away at the first crack in the surface.

And in those relationships, the rare, golden ones, there can be healing. There can be trust rebuilt. There can be laughter in the spaces where silence once lived.

But even if those relationships are few, your worth does not diminish because others failed to understand your illness. You are not broken. You are not unlovable. You are not the sum of the things that went wrong.

You are someone living through something unimaginably hard. You are trying, even when it doesn't look graceful. And that effort, that grit, that desperate hope for connection despite the chaos — it means something.

PMDD may have cost me people I loved. But it also taught me what real love looks like. And I am slowly learning to give that kind of love to myself, even when others can't.

Even when they leave.

Especially then.

"It wasn't that I stopped loving them. It's that I couldn't reach them from inside the storm."

5.2 Burnout & Backlash

Missed jobs, ruined dreams, exhausted bodies

There are years I don't remember properly. Just a blur of trying, failing, crashing, and recovering. Over and over again. The body gets tired. The mind gets tired. Life begins to feel like a punishment.

PMDD doesn't just live in your hormones. It creeps into every corner of your life, including the parts you once felt proud of. Work, ambition, creativity, stability. It eats away at your consistency. And in a world that worships productivity, that's often the beginning of the end.

I wanted to have a career. I had plans. I had potential. But the problem with PMDD is that you can be brilliant for half the month and barely functioning for the rest. You start strong, then disappear. You deliver something exceptional, then miss the next deadline. You impress, then implode. And over time, people stop trusting you. Not because you're not good at what you do, but because you're not reliable. That word alone becomes your enemy. Unreliable. Flaky. Moody. Difficult.

It's not laziness. It's not lack of passion. It's burnout. And not the kind that comes from overworking for years. The kind that comes from fighting your own body like clockwork, month after month. The kind where your brain feels like it's on fire, your chest is heavy with dread, and the simplest task feels impossible.

I've left jobs I loved because I couldn't keep up. I've ghosted opportunities that once excited me because I was in a fog so thick I couldn't see a future. I've watched others rise while I sat frozen, too exhausted to even try. And then came the shame. The self-blame. The long internal speeches about how I was wasting my life.

What people don't realise is how heavy the price is. Not just missed income. Not just lost promotions. But lost identity. You begin to wonder who you are if you can't be what you set out to be. You grieve the version of yourself that was going to achieve great things. You feel the sting of being left behind.

People say "just push through." But PMDD doesn't listen to pep talks. It shuts you down. It turns off the lights inside your brain. It robs you of energy, clarity, and focus. You sit staring at your to-do list and feel physically sick. You cancel interviews because you are crying on the bathroom floor. You fake sick days because "I'm suicidal before my period" doesn't sound professional.

And so your dreams gather dust.

The backlash is silent, but brutal. You fall behind on rent. You feel guilty every time you spend money. You question your worth. You can't plan ahead because you don't know how bad the next episode will be. You start choosing jobs based on flexibility, not passion. You start settling, scaling down your goals, making yourself smaller so your illness fits.

Eventually, you stop dreaming altogether. Because dreaming starts to feel like setting yourself up to fail. Hope becomes dangerous.

The physical toll is just as relentless. It's not just emotional fatigue. It's bone-deep weariness. The kind where you wake up and still feel like you haven't slept. Your muscles ache. Your skin hurts. Your digestion is out of sync. You try to exercise but feel dizzy. You try to eat well but lose your appetite. You start surviving on caffeine and silence.

Then come the medical bills. The missed appointments. The lost jobs with no sick pay. The exhaustion compounds. The healthcare system is rarely kind to women with invisible illnesses. They want you to prove it. Justify it. Explain why you are still not better. And when the tests come back "normal," you're sent home again. Tired, dismissed, and still very much unwell.

The cruellest part is watching people assume you're just not trying hard enough. They see the gaps in your CV and raise their eyebrows. They ask why you're not "doing more" with your time. They think it's about motivation. They don't see that you've been white-knuckling your way through every day just to stay afloat.

I once had a manager tell me I needed to "snap out of my funk." He said I was too sensitive. Said I should leave my personal problems at the door. I nodded. I went to the bathroom. I cried. Then I went home and didn't return the next day. Or the next.

This is what it's like to live with PMDD in a world that demands consistency. You're expected to show up, smile, and perform even when your brain is telling you to disappear. And when you can't, you pay the price. Financially. Professionally. Personally.

For many of us, our careers don't follow straight lines. They're broken into fragments, interrupted by periods of survival. We freelance because it gives us more control. We turn down promotions because the pressure would be too much. We take time off and call it "burnout," but really it's PMDD stealing another piece of our stability.

And still, we rise. Maybe not as quickly as others. Maybe not as smoothly. But we do. We adapt. We learn to work in cycles. We build soft routines that honour our energy levels. We create spaces where we don't have to pretend. We find purpose in new places, even if they look different from what we imagined.

Some days, I mourn the dreams I couldn't follow. I feel the ache of a life interrupted. But I also recognise the strength it takes to keep going in a body that is constantly betraying you. To keep trying. To keep showing up, even when the world doesn't understand the battle.

This is not weakness. This is endurance.

And maybe, just maybe, the dream now is survival with dignity. Stability without shame. A life that honours the rhythm of my body, rather than punishes it.

PMDD may have derailed my plans. But I am still here. Still building. Still finding meaning.

5.3 Forgiving Yourself
Letting go of guilt for things you didn't choose

No one tells you how hard it will be to forgive yourself for something that was never your fault. That's the quiet cruelty of PMDD. The symptoms hurt, yes. The fallout is real. But the guilt is the part that lingers long after the worst days have passed. It burrows deep. It whispers that everything that went wrong was somehow your doing.

There is guilt for the things you said. The things you didn't say. The days you missed. The people you pushed away. The moments when you lost control. The hours when you disappeared into the fog and left people wondering where you had gone. You feel the weight of it in your chest, like a stone you carry from room to room, from month to month.

Sometimes it is sharp and specific. You remember a birthday ruined by an episode. A partner who stopped trying to understand. A deadline missed because you couldn't get out of bed. And other times, it is vague but constant. A hum in the background of your life. A low-level shame that tells you that you are always letting someone down.

You try to explain it. You say, "I wasn't myself." You say, "I was in the storm." And sometimes they forgive you. But even when they do, the hardest part remains: forgiving yourself.

Because you were there. You watched it happen. You felt the anger rise, even as you told yourself to stay calm. You heard the sharpness in your voice. You saw yourself cancel, again. You watched time pass through a haze while the rest of the world kept moving.

It's hard to separate yourself from the illness when it lives inside your body. It wears your face. It uses your voice. So when it breaks things, it feels like *you* broke them.

But you didn't choose this. That's the part you must hold on to, even when everything else feels lost. You did not wake up one day and decide to be erratic. You did not decide to bleed out your joy every month. You did not ask for your brain to become a battlefield. This happened *to* you.

Still, the mind is cruel. It plays back the worst moments like a reel on repeat. It shows you the texts you shouldn't have sent. The expression on your child's face. The project you abandoned. The apology you owe, again. It convinces you that you are the villain in your own life story.

But there is another truth, one that sits quietly beneath the noise: you are doing the best you can. Even when it looks messy. Even when you fall short. Even when your best does not meet the standards of a world that does not understand what it takes to simply survive.

Forgiveness doesn't come in a single moment. It is not a dramatic epiphany. It is slow, often painful. It happens in fragments. A small kindness to yourself on a day when you feel undeserving. A decision not to punish yourself for needing rest. A breath taken before the self-criticism lands.

It is choosing, again and again, to believe that you are more than your hardest days.

And yet, grieving is part of it too. You must grieve what PMDD has taken. Not just relationships and routines, but your own trust in yourself. The version of you who didn't fear her own mind. The one who could make plans without wondering if she would be well enough to follow through.

You are allowed to mourn the things you couldn't hold onto. You are allowed to cry for the days lost to darkness. That is not weakness. It is part of the healing.

Some days, I sit with the sadness. I let it rise. I name the things I carry: guilt for yelling at someone I love, guilt for not showing up, guilt for disappearing when someone needed me. And then I remind myself: I was unwell. I was in pain. I did not choose this.

There is something radical about turning toward yourself with compassion instead of criticism. About looking at your history and saying, "I didn't deserve what happened to me." It is not a way of avoiding responsibility. It is a way of holding space for the whole truth.

Yes, I said things I regret. But I was suffering.

Yes, I've let people down. But I was fighting to hold myself together.

Yes, I could have handled things better. But I didn't know then what I know now.

Forgiveness is not forgetting. It is remembering with tenderness.

You do not have to keep punishing yourself to prove that you care. You do not have to keep bleeding to earn the right to heal. You do not have to hold your past like a prison sentence.

You are not broken beyond repair.

You are someone who lived through something invisible and brutal, again and again, and is still here. Still trying. Still learning. Still choosing to believe in the possibility of peace.

"You didn't choose this. You don't have to carry the guilt as if you did."

PART

Six

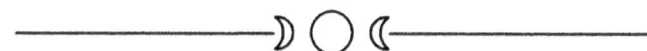

The Search for a Name

6.1 The Lost Years

All the Time Spent Not Knowing What It Was

You don't realize you're living in a mystery until someone finally gives it a name.

For years, I was the main character in a story I didn't understand. My days felt borrowed, my emotions foreign. There was a rhythm to the chaos, but I couldn't hear the beat. Some months I would feel strong and capable. Other months, always the same part of the month, I would collapse into someone I didn't recognize. I would cry until my chest hurt, lash out at the people I loved, or stare into the dark for hours, feeling like I was unravelling.

It never made sense. Not in a way anyone could pin down. And certainly not in a way anyone else took seriously.

I went to doctors. I went to therapists. I went to friends. I scoured Google searches late at night with trembling fingers, typing things like "why do I get suicidal before my period" and "rage before period normal?" And over and over again, I was handed the same answers: stress. Depression. Anxiety. Maybe PMS. Maybe nothing. Maybe I was just too sensitive. Maybe I was imagining it.

But I wasn't imagining the patterns.

Every month, for at least ten days, I would become someone else. I was terrified of her. She hated the world. She hated herself. She didn't want to be here. And then the bleed would come, and just like that, she would vanish. I'd return to myself, blinking in the aftermath like someone waking from a fever dream. The guilt, the confusion, the shame would remain, but the rage and despair would loosen their grip, for a while.

This went on for years.

I lost time. So much time. Whole seasons passed in a fog of survival. I dropped out of things I loved. I ended relationships I couldn't hold onto. I burned bridges I couldn't explain. I apologized constantly but didn't know for what. I thought I was broken. I thought I was cursed. I thought I was beyond repair.

Looking back, I now understand what was happening. But back then, I was living inside it. You can't map a storm while you're drowning in it.

What made it harder was how easily the world brushed it off. I can't count the number of times I tried to speak about what was happening, only to be met with a chuckle or a shrug. "Hormones," people said, as though that explained the way I would lie on the bathroom floor sobbing, or consider ending everything just to make the pain stop. "Everyone gets a bit moody before their period." But this wasn't moodiness. It was a full-scale possession. It was life-ruining.

I was 28 when I first stumbled across the acronym PMDD. I remember the moment with eerie clarity. I wasn't even looking for it. I had spiralled into yet another episode, desperate and alone, and found myself on an obscure message board. A woman was describing something that sounded exactly like me, how she would scream at her partner then collapse in grief, how she couldn't stand to be in her own skin, how she felt normal again the moment her period began. She called it PMDD. Premenstrual Dysphoric Disorder.

I had never heard of it.

I clicked. I read. I devoured. My entire life began rearranging itself around the possibility of this truth. The symptoms matched. The cycle matched. The desperation, the chaos, the two selves—it all matched. There was a term. There was research. There were other people. I wasn't alone. And most importantly, I wasn't crazy.

However with that relief came something else: grief. Deep, aching grief. Because suddenly, I could see just how many years I had spent not knowing. How much time I had wasted blaming myself. How many decisions had been made under the shadow of something I didn't understand. It was like turning on the light after years of stumbling through a dark room, only to see the bruises on your shins and arms and wonder how much pain could have been avoided if someone had just handed you the switch.

The lost years were real. They were formative. They shaped my sense of self in ways I'm still untangling. When you spend a decade believing you're unstable, dramatic, or difficult, it leaves marks. Even now, with a diagnosis and a name and a community, I still struggle to trust myself. I second-guess my emotions. I fear the return of the other version of me. I carry the weight of those misdiagnosed years like stones in my pockets.

I think this is something many people with PMDD face: the devastation of not knowing. It's not just about the suffering. It's about the silence that surrounds it. The way medical systems overlook it. The way families minimize it. The way even we, the ones living it, start to doubt our own reality. Because if it were real, someone would have seen it, right? If it were real, someone would have named it sooner.

That's the betrayal. That's the wound.

It's not just that I was sick. It's that I was sick and invisible.

I often think about who I might have been if I had known sooner. What might I have achieved? Who might I have saved—especially myself? It's a cruel thing, to wonder how different your life could have been if the world had just handed you the right words at the right time.

And yet, I also know this: I'm not alone. There are thousands of us walking out of the fog with new vocabulary, new understanding, and new clarity. We are reclaiming our stories. We are piecing together our pasts with the compassion they always deserved. We are finding each other, and in doing so, we are finding the parts of ourselves we thought were lost.

There is power in naming. There is power in knowing. But there is also pain in the realization of how long you lived without it. Those lost years matter. They are part of the story. They are part of the wound. But they are also the beginning of the fight—for answers, for healing, for recognition.

We deserved better. And now, we're demanding it.

"Not knowing what was wrong didn't mean nothing was. It just meant the world hadn't caught up to your pain yet."

6.2 Finding the Pattern

That Moment You Start Tracking and Suspect the Cycle

It begins as a hunch. A question in the back of your mind that says, *haven't we been here before?*

There is something eerily familiar about the feelings. The rage that bubbles up without warning. The grief that swallows you whole. The anxiety that coils in your stomach like a tightening rope. They always seem to arrive when your life is going well, and they always seem to leave just as abruptly. You start to feel like a fraud in your own mind. Why am I like this? Why can't I hold it together?

And then one day, somewhere between another emotional fallout and the guilt-drenched cleanup, the question sharpens. *Could this be hormonal?*

At first, it feels too easy. Too obvious. You've spent so long searching for explanations that it almost feels foolish to consider your menstrual cycle might be involved. You've been told hormones can make you a bit snappy, maybe tired, a little bloated. But suicidal? Enraged? Like a danger to yourself? That can't be normal. That must mean something else is wrong with you.

Still, the doubt lingers.

So you start watching. Quietly. You begin to track your symptoms, maybe with an app or a calendar, maybe just scribbled notes in the margins of a planner. You don't tell anyone. You're not even sure you believe yourself yet. You just begin to observe. The tracking isn't scientific. It's desperate. You are collecting clues from the crime scene of your own life.

Day 18: Woke up crying. Snapped at Mum. Hate myself.
Day 19: Couldn't get out of bed. Thoughts again.
Day 22: Feel like I'm losing it. Everything hurts.
Day 26: Period came. Everything suddenly fine. What the hell?

You flip back through weeks. Then months. The same pattern starts to emerge. The dip always comes at the same time. A week or so before your period. The same spirals. The same arguments. The same isolation. You weren't imagining it. It wasn't random. It was timed. Regular. Predictable, even. And that realization shakes something loose in you.

This is not a personality flaw. This is not just anxiety. You are not unstable all the time. You are being hijacked. On a schedule.

It is a strange feeling, the first time you connect the dots. You feel validated and betrayed all at once. Validated, because you knew something wasn't right. Betrayed, because no one told you to look at your cycle sooner. All the doctors you saw. All the sessions you cried through. All the pills you were given. Why didn't anyone suggest tracking?

You might feel foolish for not noticing it earlier. But how could you? You were inside the storm, trying to survive it. You were told not to make a fuss about hormones. You were told to calm down, to be reasonable, to not overreact. You were told it was stress. Maybe trauma. Maybe you just needed to work harder at self-care.

But now you have data. You have evidence. You have a recurring map of the emotional devastation that lines up with your biology. And that is terrifying. Because if your brain and body can betray you like this every month, what does that mean? What does that say about your future? About your sense of self?

Still, there's a strange comfort in the discovery. There's structure in the madness. You stop thinking of yourself as completely broken. You start thinking of yourself as someone who has something happening *to* them. Not someone who *is* something wrong.

This is often the turning point.

You begin to warn people. "I think something's going on with my hormones." You start to plan your life around the storm. You try to schedule less in the danger window. You start learning the vocabulary. Luteal phase. Estrogen drop. Progesterone sensitivity. The words are clunky in your mouth, but they give shape to the thing that has haunted you. They are small weapons against the darkness.

You might start reading forums. Finding others. Swapping stories. You begin to see yourself reflected back. The same stories. The same patterns. The same desperate questions. The same exhausted relief. It's not just you.

For many, this is also when the self-blame starts to unravel. You forgive yourself for the missed birthdays, the burned-out jobs, the friendships that couldn't survive the storm. You start to say things like "I wasn't well then" instead of "I'm a terrible person." You still feel the guilt, but now it has a context. Now it has a name.

You may not have an official diagnosis yet, but that moment you first track the pattern is when something shifts. It is the beginning of reclaiming your story. Of seeing yourself clearly. Of understanding that you are not the villain—you are the witness, the survivor, the one who kept going even without answers.

It's not everything. But it's the start. And sometimes, the start is what saves you.

6.3 When You Finally Know

Diagnosis: Relief, Grief, Fear, and Validation

There is a moment when it all clicks into place.

For some, it comes in a doctor's office. For others, it happens alone, at 3 a.m., reading an article that explains your entire life back to you. Whether it's a clinical diagnosis or self-discovery, it carries the weight of something enormous. You finally know. It has a name. PMDD. Premenstrual Dysphoric Disorder.

Those four letters can change everything. But they don't come quietly.

At first, there's the flood of relief. A fierce, almost dizzying validation. You weren't imagining it. You weren't being dramatic. You weren't weak, hysterical, or ungrateful. You were living with a severe, hormone-related disorder that was hijacking your brain and your body with surgical precision, month after month. What happened to you had a pattern, a mechanism, a scientific explanation. You cry, not because you're sad, but because someone finally turned on the lights. After years in the dark, you finally see the shape of the thing you've been fighting.

Relief is just the beginning…

Almost immediately, the grief rolls in behind it. Quiet and sharp. It touches everything. All the years you didn't know. All the people you hurt. The friends who pulled away. The relationships that couldn't survive it. The jobs you lost, the opportunities you missed, the self-esteem you buried just to keep going. You start to count the wreckage, and it's a long list.

You think back to your younger self and feel a tenderness that almost breaks you. She wasn't out of control. She wasn't a mess. She was in pain. She was fighting a monster with no name. And no one helped her.

You may even find yourself grieving a version of life that could have been. What would have happened if you had been diagnosed earlier? How much harm could have been avoided? How many years could have been different if someone, anyone, had just connected the dots for you?

Then comes the fear.

Diagnosis does not come with a cure. There is no simple fix, no one-size-fits-all solution. You quickly realize that having a name doesn't mean you get to hand the pain back. It's still yours. Now it just has paperwork.

And with that paperwork comes uncertainty. What now? Will people take this seriously? Will your doctor know what to do? Will your friends understand? How much of your life has to change to make space for this condition?

You might begin to notice how little awareness there still is around PMDD. How even medical professionals seem unfamiliar with it.

How much you are still expected to explain, to advocate, to prove. It is exhausting to be newly diagnosed and still not believed. To know exactly what's wrong, but still be met with silence, confusion, or worse, dismissal.

And yet, there is so much power in knowledge.

The diagnosis becomes an anchor. A way to chart your experience. A tool to separate yourself from the storm. You stop saying "I'm going crazy" and start saying "my luteal phase has started." You stop drowning in shame and start learning how to prepare, how to manage, how to speak about it with clarity. You become your own translator, turning pain into language, language into strategy.

The more you learn, the more connected you feel. You find others who have been through the same thing. You share symptoms, medications, supplements, side effects, survival tips. You discover that PMDD is not rare—but it is underdiagnosed, under-researched, and deeply misunderstood. The loneliness begins to crack. You find community in the unspoken. You find solidarity in the recognition.

There is something bittersweet about this stage. You have more tools, but also more questions. You have more words, but also more responsibility. You are no longer invisible, but you are not yet safe. It is the beginning of a long road, not just toward treatment, but toward healing the wounds of the time you spent not knowing.

And the truth is, knowing changes your relationship with yourself.

You begin to reframe your past, seeing it not as a personal failure but as a medical history. You forgive yourself, slowly. You learn to monitor, to adapt. You build systems of care that weren't there before. You teach people around you what PMDD is, even as you're still figuring it out yourself. You become both patient and advocate. You carry your diagnosis like a torch and a burden.

But most importantly, you begin to trust yourself again.

That's the quiet miracle. After years of second-guessing your instincts, doubting your own reality, and blaming yourself for what you couldn't control, the diagnosis says *you were right*. Your body was trying to tell you something. You were not overreacting. You were surviving. You were right to ask questions. You were right to keep searching.

You were always right to believe that something wasn't right.

And now, you know.

PART

Seven

The Medical Shrug

Chapter 7.1: The Doctor Gauntlet

Scripts, Referrals, Miscommunication

You've finally realised there's a pattern. You've tracked your moods for months. You've written down the days when the world caves in and the days when it lifts again. You're not just imagining this. You're not just "emotional." There's a cycle. You feel both vindicated and terrified.

So, you do what we're told to do. You make an appointment.

The first doctor is kind but distracted. They nod as you explain the crashes that come monthly. They type something into a screen while you speak about suicidal thoughts that seem to evaporate when your period arrives. You mention rage. Insomnia. Bloating. Dissociation. Crying in the bathroom at work, then pretending nothing happened.

They offer you an antidepressant. Maybe Sertraline. Maybe Fluoxetine. They say it might help. You ask if it's PMDD. They say they're not sure. "Could be hormonal. Could be depression. Either way, SSRIs can be effective." They print a script and hand it to you like a bus ticket. You leave with questions buzzing like flies in your head.

You take the pills. Maybe they help. Maybe they don't. Maybe they numb you so much you can't feel anything at all. Or maybe you feel a slight lift, but the luteal crash still comes. The violent mood drop. The impossible heaviness. The part of you that can't be reached.

So, you go back.

This time, you ask for a referral. You've read about specialists online. Maybe a gynaecologist. Maybe a psychiatrist. You're not sure which route is best, because PMDD sits in the no-man's land between physical and mental health. The receptionist doesn't know either. She raises her eyebrows at your question. She asks, "So, is this for anxiety or periods?" You say both. She frowns and tells you to book a double appointment next time.

You're referred to genecology. It takes three months. You wait. You bleed. You crash. You rise. You crash again. Life keeps happening, and you keep surviving it.

The gynaecologist looks at your chart. She glances at your notes. "PMDD?" she says, like it's an unfamiliar acronym. "Well, we don't diagnose that here. That's more psychiatric." You try to explain that it is hormone-related. That it's in the DSM-5. That you've done the tracking. That you've researched treatments. She sighs and says, "Maybe try the pill."

You've already tried the pill.

You've tried the pill that made your hair fall out. The one that turned you into a zombie. The one that made you bleed for weeks. The one that helped for two months and then stopped helping altogether. You tell her this. She writes it down, nods slowly, and says, "Sometimes it's trial and error."

You are so tired of being an error.

Next comes the psychiatrist. It takes another referral. Another wait. Another month where you beg your partner not to leave you. Another month where you cry over nothing and snap over everything. The psychiatrist tells you PMDD is a "controversial diagnosis." They mention borderline personality disorder. They ask about childhood trauma. They suggest CBT. You ask about hormonal treatments. They say that's not their area. You're passed back to gynaecology. Again.

It becomes a game of hot potato with your body. A volley between departments, none of which want to take ownership. You start to feel like a difficult patient. You start to wonder if you *are* difficult. If you're exaggerating. If it's really all in your head.

But then your period arrives, and the fog lifts, and you remember who you are. You *know* something is wrong.

So, you try private clinics. You email specialists. You sit on waiting lists. You ask for hormone level testing and are told that levels fluctuate too much for tests to be meaningful. You request a hysterectomy and are told you're too young, or might change your mind, or "let's try a few more options first." You're bounced from gynaecology to endocrinology to mental health services. You chase answers while managing a body that betrays you once a month with surgical precision.

And each time, you're expected to advocate for yourself. Calmly. Professionally. Without emotion. Without frustration. Even when the thing you are fighting for is your sanity.

This is the medical gauntlet. You run it with a mix of rage and resilience. You learn the language of referrals and discharge summaries. You carry a folder of symptom charts and treatment notes. You get good at explaining PMDD in thirty seconds or less, with zero room for doubt in your voice.

Sometimes you get lucky. A nurse nods in recognition. A GP looks you in the eye and says, "I believe you." A specialist takes your history seriously. These moments are gold. They can change everything.

But too often, what you get instead is the shrug.

The shrug that says "I don't know."
The shrug that means "It's not my job."
The shrug that puts it all back on you.

And that shrug? It is not benign. It's a quiet dismissal that sends you spiralling back into despair. Because what you're really asking is: *Please help me not lose myself again next month.* What you hear instead is: *You'll have to figure this out alone.*

But let's be constructive.

This isn't about blaming every doctor. Many of them are overworked. Many want to help. The problem is systemic. PMDD lives in the cracks between disciplines. It's poorly taught, poorly researched, poorly prioritised. There are no clear treatment pathways. No standardised care plans. Many medical professionals have never even heard of it.

We need cross-specialty collaboration. We need training. We need funding for research, and proper guidelines for diagnosis and treatment. We need to stop pushing patients through a maze of appointments that lead nowhere. We need doctors who can say, "I don't know, but I'll find out."

Until then, patients will keep surviving in limbo.

We'll keep showing up, exhausted but determined. We'll keep explaining ourselves, over and over. We'll keep hoping the next door we knock on leads to someone who sees us.

Because at the end of the day, that's all we're asking for.

To be seen. To be heard. To be helped.
Before the cycle begins again.

Chapter 7.2: How to Advocate for Yourself
Tips for Getting Heard

You walk into the room with your notes. You've rehearsed what to say. You've been up all night reading about GnRH agonists, SSRIs, and the luteal phase. You've tracked your symptoms for months, maybe years. But the moment you sit down and the doctor asks, "So, how can I help today?", your mind blanks. You feel small. Unsure. You lose your footing, even though you've lived every second of this battle.

Advocating for yourself in a medical setting is not something we're taught. Especially not when we're women. Especially not when our symptoms are "emotional." Especially not when we are sobbing and shaking and terrified that we're about to be misunderstood all over again.

No one is more qualified to speak about your body than you.

No one else has lived through your worst days. No one else has tried to keep working, parenting, functioning, while your brain told you the world was ending. You may not have a medical degree, but you have the lived experience, and that matters.

So how do you get heard when the system is stacked against you? How do you stay standing when the appointment is rushed, or the specialist looks at you like you're dramatic, hormonal, or "just stressed"?

Here are the tools I've learned, built, and borrowed along the way. Not perfect. Not foolproof. But battle-tested.

Track, Track, Track

This is your primary evidence. Not vague memories. Not feelings. But hard data.

Start a symptom tracker. Use an app, a spreadsheet, or even a notebook. Track every day of your cycle, emotions, physical symptoms, sleep, energy, suicidal thoughts, rage, cravings, anything. Include the day of your period. Use it to spot patterns. PMDD is cyclical. A pattern over three consecutive cycles is powerful.

Bring this data to your appointments. It turns "I feel awful" into "Here's a documented pattern of severe symptoms that resolve shortly after menstruation." That's the language the system understands.

Write a Script Before Your Appointment

It's easy to forget things in the room. Appointments can feel intimidating, especially if you're already mentally depleted.

Write out what you want to say. Literally. Bullet points. A paragraph. A script. Include:

- A summary of your symptoms
- How they affect your life
- Your cycle tracking data

- What you've already tried

- What you're hoping for (e.g., a diagnosis, a treatment, a referral)

You can even hand this to the doctor at the beginning of the appointment. It helps steer the conversation and shows you've done your homework.

Name the Condition

Say the words. *Premenstrual Dysphoric Disorder.*

Not "PMS." Not "I get emotional before my period." Call it what it is. If the doctor isn't familiar, briefly explain: "It's a hormone sensitivity disorder. It's in the DSM-5. It affects mood and functioning severely in the luteal phase."

Speaking the name helps break the silence that still surrounds PMDD. It places it in medical language. It signals you know what you're talking about.

Bring Backup

Bring a friend, partner, or advocate if you can. Someone who has seen your symptoms. Someone who can say, "This isn't just moodiness. I've seen her disappear. I've seen her in crisis."

If that's not possible, bring a written statement from someone who's witnessed it. A partner, a friend, even a note from a therapist. External voices can lend credibility when yours feels fragile.

Ask for Specific Next Steps

Don't leave the room empty-handed. Before the appointment ends, ask clearly:

- Can you refer me to a gynaecologist/psychiatrist who understands PMDD?

- Can we trial hormonal treatment or cycle-specific SSRIs?

- Are there other diagnostic steps we can take?

Be clear that you want follow-up. Ask when you'll be contacted. Ask what you should do if the treatment doesn't help. Don't let it float into the void.

Know Your Rights

You are allowed to:

- Ask for a second opinion

- Request a referral

- Decline a treatment that hasn't worked before

- Have access to your medical records

- Make a complaint if you are dismissed or mistreated

The healthcare system may be flawed, but you are not powerless in it. You are a patient, not a problem.

Use Keywords That Get Noticed

Certain words set off alarm bells in the right way. They indicate severity and help you get taken seriously. These include:

- *Suicidal ideation*

- *Severe impairment of daily functioning*

- *Cyclical pattern*

- *DSM-5 recognised condition*

- *Hormone sensitivity disorder*

These are not exaggerations. They are accurate descriptors of what many people with PMDD go through.

If You Don't Get Help, Don't Stop

If a doctor dismisses you, do not let that become the story.

Try another. And another.

Yes, it is exhausting. It shouldn't be like this. You should not have to fight. But until the system catches up, persistence becomes your lifeline. Your story matters. You are not overreacting. You are not difficult. You are navigating a broken map with no guide, and every step forward counts.

Connect with the PMDD Community

You don't have to do this alone. There are online support groups. There are forums, charities, and social media communities filled with people who *get it*. They can recommend doctors. Share template letters. Help you prepare for appointments. Validate what you've lived through.

Find your people. They will help you stay strong on the days you feel like giving up.

Keep the Focus on Functioning

When describing symptoms, shift the focus to how it affects your life:

- "I miss work every month because I'm non-functional in the week before my period."

- "I have suicidal thoughts that go away as soon as I bleed."

- "I'm scared of what I might do in the luteal phase."

- "This is destroying my ability to maintain relationships."

This isn't about "feeling emotional." It's about losing control of your life for two weeks every month. Make that clear.

The Bottom Line

You should not have to fight this hard to be believed. You should not have to walk into every appointment ready for battle. But right now, for many of us, that is the reality.

So, when you can, when you have the strength, advocate. Loudly or quietly. In writing or in person. Through tears or with fire in your voice. However you can.

Because every time you speak the words, you are changing something. In yourself. In your care. In the system, slowly.

You are not "just hormonal." You are not "too sensitive." You are a person living with a serious condition that deserves attention, treatment, and compassion. And you have every right to be heard.

PART

Eight

Hormones 101

8.1 The Hormone Cycle Demystified

Progesterone, Estrogen, Luteal Shifts

If you've ever tried to understand what's going on inside your body during PMDD, chances are you ended up overwhelmed or underwhelmed. Either the information was buried in clinical jargon, or it was brushed off with vague phrases like "hormonal changes." But the truth is, there's a real and intricate chemical story unfolding inside you every month, and once you start to grasp it, things that once felt random start to make a strange kind of sense.

At the centre of the hormone horror show there are two major players: estrogen and progesterone. These are the main messengers behind the scenes, running a complex biological relay race throughout your cycle. They are not the enemy. But for some people, particularly those with PMDD, the way the brain responds to these hormones can trigger profound emotional and physical shifts that go far beyond the usual premenstrual experience.

Let's talk science. Estrogen is often seen as the more energizing hormone. It builds gradually and helps your brain produce serotonin; the chemical most commonly associated with mood, motivation, and a general sense of wellbeing. When estrogen is rising, many people feel brighter, more social, more mentally clear. It's the hormone that often makes you feel like you're "back to yourself" after a rough patch. But estrogen doesn't stay stable. It fluctuates throughout the cycle, and in PMDD, even small dips can feel like cliffs. A gentle drop in estrogen, which wouldn't be a big deal for most people, can lead to a sudden, jarring slide into anxiety, fogginess, or low mood in someone with PMDD.

Progesterone enters the scene after ovulation and becomes the dominant hormone in the second half of the cycle. In theory, progesterone is calming. It's meant to soothe the system, help you rest, and support emotional steadiness as the body prepares for a potential pregnancy. But if you have PMDD, your brain may not process progesterone the way it's supposed to. In fact, it's not the hormone itself that causes problems, but a specific byproduct of it: a neurosteroid called allopregnanolone.

Allopregnanolone, or ALLO, is derived from progesterone and affects GABA receptors in the brain. GABA is your brain's natural calming chemical. It slows down neural activity and helps you feel peaceful and regulated. For most people, ALLO boosts GABA's effects and promotes relaxation. But in PMDD, the brain may become overly sensitive or oddly resistant to ALLO. The result can feel like emotional whiplash, where calm suddenly turns to chaos without any external cause.

This sensitivity is what makes PMDD so hard to live with. The hormone levels themselves are usually within the normal range. There's no imbalance on paper. But your brain's *response* to those normal fluctuations is not typical. That's why it's not as simple as "you just have PMS" or "your hormones are a bit off." PMDD is a neuroendocrine condition, meaning it's a problem in how the brain and hormones interact. The signals get scrambled. The same substances that might soothe one person can trigger panic, rage, or despair in another.

And then, just as mysteriously as it began, it ends. Hormone levels shift again. The storm passes. You wake up one day and feel like you've returned to yourself, clear, stable, functional. This is often the most confusing part. The contrast is so stark, it can leave you questioning your own sanity. How could yesterday you have been lying on the floor crying and today you're answering emails and making jokes? The answer lies in those chemical messengers, especially the drop-off of progesterone and ALLO, and the return of estrogen to your system. When these hormones reset, so does your mind.

Understanding the mechanics of these shifts doesn't make the experience less painful. But it does offer a framework. It reminds you that this isn't your fault. You are not unstable. You are responding to powerful forces in your body that most people, including doctors, barely understand. For decades, PMDD was either misdiagnosed as a mood disorder or dismissed entirely. But research is finally catching up. Scientists are beginning to map out the genetic, neurological, and hormonal patterns that define this condition, and they're discovering that it's not about willpower, weakness, or personality. It's about sensitivity. Not emotional sensitivity, but biological sensitivity. A nervous system that reacts fiercely to hormonal cues.

What's even more fascinating is that PMDD doesn't show up when estrogen or progesterone are artificially high or low in isolation. It emerges in the presence of *fluctuation*. It's the changes that seem to trigger symptoms, not the steady presence of the hormone itself. That's why some people find relief when hormone levels are suppressed or stabilized through medication or menopause. It's not about removing the hormones, but about avoiding the rollercoaster.

That rollercoaster is not just steep, it's unpredictable. You might have a few months where the luteal shift feels manageable, and then suddenly, for reasons unknown, you're back in the thick of it, watching your personality unravel. It can be hard to trust your body when it behaves like this. But by learning the chemical choreography behind the curtain, you can begin to separate *you* from the symptoms. You can start to chart the rhythms, notice the early tremors, and build plans around the inevitable shifts.

No one chooses to live with a body that turns into a stranger. But knowledge is a form of power. Knowing that there is a pattern, a real, measurable, hormonal cycle, behind your worst days can be the first step in reclaiming some sense of agency. You might not be able to stop the tides, but you can learn when they're coming. And sometimes, that's enough to start swimming instead of drowning.

8.2 PMDD and the Brain

Serotonin Sensitivity, Mood Regulation, and Chaos

Let's talk about the brain. Not just the brain as an organ, but the brain as your internal command centre, the place where your thoughts, emotions, behaviours, and reactions are born, filtered, and managed. In PMDD, this command centre goes into disarray. And although the condition is linked to hormonal shifts, the real chaos happens inside the brain itself.

People often misunderstand PMDD as a hormonal imbalance. But that's not quite accurate. What makes PMDD different is not the levels of hormones in your body, but how your brain *responds* to them. And that response is deeply wired into your brain chemistry, especially the system that handles mood regulation.

One of the key players in this process is serotonin, a neurotransmitter that helps control mood, sleep, appetite, memory, and even pain perception. It's often referred to as the brain's "feel-good chemical," but that description doesn't capture how essential it really is. Serotonin is more like a stabiliser. It doesn't just lift your mood, it keeps your inner weather system from becoming a hurricane.

In people with PMDD, this serotonin system seems to work differently. Researchers believe that the brain becomes unusually sensitive to fluctuations in certain hormones, particularly during the second half of the menstrual cycle. But what makes that sensitivity so destabilising is that it disrupts serotonin signalling. The brain starts having trouble making, releasing, or responding to serotonin at the very moment it's needed most.

This serotonin disruption doesn't look like a small emotional wobble. It can feel like a total collapse of your ability to regulate mood. One moment you're calm. The next, you're crying over a cereal advert or snapping at someone for breathing too loudly. You may not feel in control of your reactions, and that's because, on a neurological level, you *aren't*. Your emotional brakes have gone offline.

It's not just mood swings either. Serotonin also affects how you process stress. When the serotonin system is functioning well, it acts like a cushion, it helps you absorb pressure without breaking. But when that system falters, small frustrations become overwhelming. The normal background noise of life starts to feel unbearable. You might feel unsafe in your own skin, panicked by things you can't name, or utterly flattened by simple tasks.

Another way this shows up is in the brain's threat system, the part responsible for detecting danger and launching a response. In PMDD, this system can go into hyperdrive. The brain starts interpreting minor stressors as major threats. A forgotten text message feels like rejection. A missed train feels like disaster. The reaction isn't dramatic for attention. It's automatic. Your brain is operating as if the world has suddenly become a more dangerous place.

And because serotonin also plays a role in memory and cognitive function, the luteal phase can bring fog, indecision, and detachment. You may find it hard to recall what you said yesterday or struggle to finish a thought. Some people describe this as watching their own life from behind a glass wall. The lights are on, but they're flickering. The words don't come out right. Everything feels disconnected, surreal, or numb.

Perhaps one of the cruellest features of this shift is that it doesn't just affect how you *feel*, it affects how you *think about yourself*. When your brain isn't producing or using serotonin properly, your inner narrative can turn dark. Not because your life has changed, but because the filter through which you see it has. You start believing things that aren't true, that you're a burden, a failure, unlovable, too much, not enough. These thoughts can spiral quickly, and it can be incredibly difficult to argue with them from the inside.

This is not a character flaw. It's a chemical lens. When the serotonin system is functioning poorly, it colours your perception of everything, including yourself. What makes PMDD especially devastating is that this altered perception doesn't just last for a few hours, it can take over half your month. And when the fog lifts, you're left picking up the pieces, wondering how your mind betrayed you so completely.

It's important to know that PMDD is increasingly being recognised as a neurobiological disorder, a condition where the structure and chemistry of the brain itself are uniquely sensitive to hormonal cues. Brain imaging studies have found differences in activity in areas that handle emotional regulation, impulse control, and memory. These aren't dramatic abnormalities, but subtle differences that, when triggered by hormonal shifts, create very real suffering.

Some of the most common misdiagnoses for PMDD, major depression, anxiety, borderline personality disorder, happen because these brain symptoms are so intense, they mimic those other conditions. But what sets PMDD apart is the *rhythmic pattern* of chaos. It comes. It goes. It returns. Always in sync with your cycle. And this pattern points not just to the body, but to the brain's inability to maintain stability under hormonal stress.

There's no quick fix for a brain that reacts like this. But there *is* hope in understanding it. The more we learn about serotonin sensitivity and PMDD, the closer we get to treatments that work — ones that go beyond sedating the body and instead help stabilise the brain's natural rhythms.

For many, this includes SSRIs (medications that enhance serotonin signalling), cognitive therapies that strengthen emotional resilience, and cycle tracking that helps you anticipate the shifts before they hit. But even without a perfect solution, there is power in knowledge. There is relief in naming the storm for what it is, not a failure of character, but a neurological response to a cycle that moves through you like a tide.

8.3 Why PMDD Happens

Genetics, Trauma, and Triggers

When you live with PMDD, it's hard not to ask *why*. Why is this happening to me? Why can't I cope the way others do? Why do I fall apart while the world keeps turning?

It's a natural question. But it's often met with unsatisfying answers, or worse, with silence. For years, PMDD was treated as a mystery illness. And when the science doesn't step up to explain suffering, shame tends to fill the gap. PMDD doesn't happen because you're weak. It doesn't happen because you're unstable or dramatic. There are real reasons. And none of them are your fault.

Let's start with genetics. One of the most promising areas of research in PMDD is the idea of genetic sensitivity. Scientists have found that people with PMDD may have subtle differences in how certain genes function, especially genes related to the way cells respond to hormones. These genes don't cause PMDD directly. Instead, they shape how your cells react to the normal hormonal shifts that happen every month.

Think of it like a radio. Most people's radios are tuned to pick up hormonal signals at a steady volume. But in PMDD, your settings are more sensitive. The same signal comes through, but it's amplified, distorted, or scrambled. This makes the whole experience more intense, even though the input, your hormone levels, might be totally ordinary. You didn't choose these settings. They were handed to you, written into your DNA before you were even born.

Genes are only part of the story. There's growing evidence that early life experiences can also shape how your body and brain respond to stress, including hormonal stress. People who have lived through trauma, especially emotional neglect, chronic stress, or unstable environments, often develop nervous systems that are more reactive. Not broken, just highly tuned to threat and change. This doesn't mean trauma causes PMDD, but it may create a foundation where PMDD is more likely to take root.

The body remembers. Experiences from childhood or adolescence can leave invisible fingerprints on your brain's development, particularly in areas that deal with safety, identity, and regulation. If your body learned early on that the world wasn't safe or predictable, it may respond more strongly to internal shifts as well. Hormonal changes, even subtle ones, can feel like another disruption, another reason to brace for impact.

There's also some indication that inflammation may play a role. This is still being studied, but researchers have found that people with PMDD sometimes show signs of a heightened immune response, even when they're not physically ill. This kind of low-level inflammation has been linked to many mood disorders and can affect how well the brain manages emotion, energy, and resilience. It may act as an invisible background pressure that makes everything feel harder to cope with.

Other possible contributors include gut health, nutrient absorption, and even sleep patterns. The body is a deeply connected system. When one part struggles, others tend to follow. It's possible that in some people, PMDD emerges not from one single cause, but from a combination of vulnerabilities. A bit of genetic sensitivity. A difficult environment. A nervous system shaped by stress. A body trying its best to adapt to a world that often doesn't make space for it.

Of course, there's the issue of triggers. These are not causes, but catalysts. Stress is a major one. Many people report that their PMDD symptoms worsen during times of life upheaval, moving house, changing jobs, caring for a sick relative, navigating relationship issues. But even smaller shifts, like changes in routine, lack of sleep, or physical illness, can push the system past its tipping point. For some, even joyful changes like pregnancy or planning a wedding can throw things off balance.

It's important to say that PMDD is *not* something you manifest by being anxious, sensitive, or emotional. Nor is it caused by failing to do enough yoga or drinking the wrong kind of herbal tea. While lifestyle can influence symptoms, it doesn't *create* the condition. PMDD lives deeper than that. In biology. In wiring. In the places medicine is still learning how to read.

This is also why traditional mental health treatments often fall short. They target mood or behaviour without addressing the cyclical nature of what's happening. It's not that your distress isn't real, it's that it follows a rhythm that needs to be understood on its own terms. PMDD is more than a collection of feelings. It's a pattern, a loop, a repeating disruption with roots in your body's chemistry and your brain's past.

And yet, even with all this knowledge, guilt often clings to people with PMDD. The guilt of not showing up. The guilt of snapping. The guilt of missing work, ruining plans, or crying in places you swore you'd hold it together. But guilt has no rightful place here. You did not invent this condition. You did not choose to be vulnerable to it. And the strength it takes to keep going, to track, to learn, to survive, is immense.

Understanding *why* PMDD happens won't make it vanish. But it can start to undo the blame that so often follows in its wake. It can remind you that this isn't your failure. It's a system behaving in ways you didn't consent to. You didn't ask for a brain that flares under pressure. You didn't ask for a body that sounds the alarm when nothing seems wrong on the outside. But this is what you've been given, and still, you persist.

If no one has ever said it plainly: this is not your fault. Whatever caused this mix of sensitivity, experience, and chemistry, it was never about personal weakness. It was about biology meeting biography in a system that wasn't designed for this much intensity. You're not broken. You're responding. You're adapting. And every time you make it through, every time you show up again after the crash, you're proving how strong that response truly is.

PART

Nine

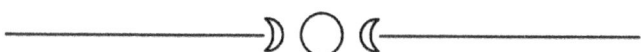

Your Toolkit of Options

9.1 Medications That Can Help

SSRIs, Birth Control, GnRH Analogues

When PMDD is disrupting your life, it can feel like the options are slim and the suffering is inevitable. But that isn't true. There *are* tools that can help. Medication may not be a magic wand, but for many, it offers a lifeline, a way to soften the edges of the monthly storm, or in some cases, prevent it entirely. It's not always a simple road, and the first thing you try might not be "the one," but there *is* a toolkit. And you have every right to reach for it.

Let's walk through the most common classes of medications used to treat PMDD. We'll look at how they work, what they might offer, and what to consider if you're thinking about trying them. This is not medical advice, but a place to get oriented before speaking with a healthcare professional who takes your symptoms seriously.

SSRIs - *Rebalancing the Mood*

Selective Serotonin Reuptake Inhibitors (SSRIs) are often the first-line treatment for PMDD. That might sound strange at first. After all, PMDD isn't a classic mood disorder. It's hormonal. So why treat it like depression?

The answer lies in how hormones like progesterone can mess with the brain's sensitivity to serotonin, a neurotransmitter involved in mood regulation, emotion, and calm. People with PMDD aren't necessarily low in serotonin. Instead, their brains seem to react differently to normal hormonal shifts, making them *feel* like they're falling into depression, anxiety, rage, or despair, even if nothing else in life has changed.

SSRIs help by making more serotonin available in the brain. They don't stop the hormone fluctuations, but they can cushion their impact. For many, this means less rage, fewer intrusive thoughts, more emotional stability, and a greater sense of control.

One of the most surprising things about SSRIs in the context of PMDD is that they don't have to be taken every day. Some people do best on continuous use, especially if their symptoms linger outside the luteal phase. Others benefit from intermittent dosing, starting the SSRI in the second half of the cycle (after ovulation) and stopping when menstruation begins. This kind of short-term, cyclical use is fairly unique to PMDD and can work well with fewer long-term side effects.

Common SSRIs used for PMDD include fluoxetine (Prozac), sertraline (Zoloft), and escitalopram (Lexapro). Side effects can include nausea, headaches, sleep disturbances, or emotional blunting, but they often fade over time. Some people find the benefits outweigh the drawbacks within just one cycle. Others need to try a few to find the right match.

What matters is this: taking an SSRI for PMDD isn't a sign of weakness or "giving up." It's a strategy, and for many, it's a powerful one.

Hormonal Birth Control - *Steadying the Shifts*

The next option is hormonal birth control. These treatments aim to *flatten* the hormonal rollercoaster that causes symptoms in the first place.

PMDD isn't caused by high or low hormones per se, but by a sensitivity to the natural *fluctuations* of estrogen and progesterone, particularly after ovulation. By using hormonal contraception to prevent ovulation and stabilize hormone levels, some people with PMDD can sidestep the monthly chaos entirely.

But not all birth control is created equal when it comes to PMDD. In fact, for some people, the wrong hormonal combination can make symptoms worse. This is often where frustration begins.

The combination pill that has shown the most promise in clinical studies is **Yaz**, which contains a unique type of progestin called drospirenone, combined with ethinyl estradiol. It's taken in a 24/4 regimen, meaning 24 active pills and only four placebo days, which helps keep hormones more consistent.

Some doctors also prescribe extended-cycle or continuous-use birth control pills, where the placebo week is skipped, and the person doesn't bleed at all for several months. This can reduce or eliminate hormonal fluctuations even further, though it doesn't work for everyone.

It's worth noting that if you've had negative experiences with hormonal birth control in the past, that doesn't mean every formulation will affect you the same way. But it's also valid to decide this route isn't for you. Some people with PMDD are particularly sensitive to synthetic hormones and feel worse, not better. That's why it's so important to work with a knowledgeable provider who listens carefully and doesn't dismiss your experiences.

GnRH Analogues - *Hitting Pause on the Cycle*

For those with severe, debilitating PMDD that hasn't responded to other treatments, GnRH analogues can offer a more aggressive option.

GnRH stands for gonadotropin-releasing hormone. Analogues of this hormone essentially tell the body to stop producing estrogen and progesterone altogether. This puts the body into a temporary, reversible menopausal state. No cycle. No ovulation. No luteal phase.

The result? For many, a dramatic reduction, or complete elimination, of PMDD symptoms.

GnRH analogues are often delivered via injection (like leuprolide) or nasal spray and are typically used short-term, often as a diagnostic trial. If symptoms disappear while on the medication, it can confirm that PMDD is the culprit. Some patients continue longer-term use, but because these medications also suppress estrogen (which is crucial for bone health, heart health, and cognitive function), they are usually paired with add-back therapy, small doses of estrogen and sometimes progesterone to protect the body while still preventing symptoms.

It's a big step, and not without risks. But for some, it is the first time in years they've felt like themselves.

What to Expect When Starting Medication

Starting any medication for PMDD can feel both hopeful and nerve-wracking. You might wonder:

Will it work?

Will I feel numb?

Will I lose parts of myself I like?

These are absolutely fair questions. Adjusting to medication can take time. Some people feel better quickly. Others need to trial several options or tweak dosages before things settle. There might be bumps along the way. That doesn't mean you're doing it wrong.

The most important thing is to have a clinician who understands PMDD and is willing to collaborate with you, not dictate to you. Someone who hears you when you say, "This isn't working," or "Something feels off." A good prescriber will help you weigh benefits and side effects, and they won't dismiss your concerns as "just hormones."

And you are allowed to change your mind. Trying a medication doesn't commit you to it for life. You can reassess. You can explore alternatives. You can say, "This helped, but I need more," or, "This made things worse, let's try something else."

Medication is one part of the toolkit, not the whole toolbox, but a vital one for many people. Choosing it isn't giving in. It's choosing yourself. It's saying, "I deserve to feel better. I deserve support. I deserve options."

Whether it's an SSRI taken during the luteal phase, a birth control pill that smooths the cycle, or a more intensive approach like GnRH analogues, these are not band-aids. They're lifelines. And every person with PMDD deserves access to them, free from shame or delay.

9.2 Therapy, Movement & Nutrition

Holistic Approaches and Their Limits

When you're living with PMDD, it's easy to fall into the trap of thinking you just haven't tried hard enough. Maybe if you cut out dairy. Maybe if you ran five times a week. Maybe if you finally mastered mindfulness or yoga or supplements. It's a seductive thought because it gives you a sense of control. But let's be clear from the start: PMDD is not your fault, and you cannot self-care your way out of it.

That said, there are holistic tools that can offer meaningful support. They may not eliminate PMDD, but they can soften its grip. They can build resilience in your system. They can hold you together when everything else is falling apart. They matter. But they are not a cure. They are scaffolding, not foundations.

Let's walk through three areas where non-medical support can help: therapy, movement, and nutrition. Not as solutions that replace medical treatment, but as complementary tools that honour the whole of who you are.

Therapy - *For the Mind Under Siege*

When people hear "therapy," they often think of talking about their childhood, or lying on a couch and venting about work. But in the context of PMDD, therapy becomes something else. It becomes a place to reckon with the two selves: the one that exists most of the month, and the one who takes over in the luteal phase. It becomes a mirror, a lighthouse, and a witness all in one.

Living with PMDD can fracture your identity. You may find yourself doing things you don't recognise, saying things you regret, or feeling emotions that seem entirely out of proportion. This constant whiplash can erode your self-esteem, make you question your sanity, and strain your relationships. Therapy provides a space to untangle all of that.

Cognitive Behavioural Therapy (CBT) has shown some evidence of benefit in managing PMDD, particularly around thought spirals and emotional regulation. But any form of talk therapy that makes space for your lived experience can be helpful. You don't need a therapist who specialises in PMDD. You need one who believes you.

Some people also benefit from trauma-informed therapy, especially if their PMDD symptoms trigger past pain or unresolved wounds. Others prefer somatic therapy, which integrates the body into the healing process, recognising that PMDD isn't just "in your head." It lives in your body, and it often strikes from there too.

Therapy won't make PMDD go away. But it can help you stay anchored. It can help you forgive yourself. It can help you build internal scaffolding so that the crash doesn't shatter you quite so completely.

Movement - *Reclaiming Your Body*

The last thing you want to hear when you're deep in PMDD is "have you tried exercising?" And yet, movement really can help. Not because it's a magic fix, but because it can gently regulate the nervous system, reduce inflammation, and support hormone metabolism.

It doesn't have to be intense. In fact, punishing workouts can make things worse, especially if you're already running on empty. What we're talking about here is supportive movement. Movement that respects where you are in your cycle. Movement that nourishes, rather than depletes.

During the follicular phase (the first half of the cycle), you may feel strong, motivated, and energised. This is often a good time for more vigorous activity: strength training, cardio, long walks, or dance. But as ovulation passes and the luteal phase begins, you might notice your energy drop and your body feel heavier, more reactive. That's when it can help to slow things down. Think restorative yoga, stretching, gentle swimming, or even just a short walk in fresh air.

Some people with PMDD find relief in rhythmic, repetitive motion, walking, cycling, swimming, because it calms the brain and provides a sense of flow. Others need grounding movement: slow, weighted, intentional. You get to experiment. You get to listen to your body without pushing it into something punishing.

What matters most is that movement becomes a *friend*, not a taskmaster. It's not about fixing your hormones. It's about helping your body feel more like home.

Nutrition - *Fuel, Not Punishment*

There's a lot of noise online about diets for PMDD. Cut sugar. Quit gluten. Eat clean. Fast. Detox. The pressure can be relentless. But beneath the fads and fearmongering, there's a quieter truth: what you eat can influence your symptoms, but it is not your fault if you can't eat "perfectly." And you do not need to become a nutritional monk to feel better.

Nutrition for PMDD isn't about restriction. It's about *support*. The goal is to give your body the tools it needs to metabolise hormones efficiently, regulate blood sugar, and stabilise mood.

Some things have shown promise in studies and lived experience. These include:

- ✓ Eating regular meals to prevent blood sugar crashes
- ✓ Prioritising protein and healthy fats, especially in the luteal phase
- ✓ Increasing magnesium-rich foods like leafy greens, nuts, seeds, and dark chocolate
- ✓ Supporting gut health with fibre and fermented foods

✓ Reducing ultra-processed foods and inflammatory additives

Some people experiment with supplements like calcium, magnesium, vitamin B6, or chasteberry. Others work with a dietitian to tailor a plan that works with their life, not against it.

But here's the most important thing: food is not a moral issue. Eating a cookie doesn't cause your rage. Having pizza won't ruin your cycle. The goal isn't perfection. It's compassion. Nourishment. Stability. And sometimes, that means soup and toast and no guilt at all.

The Limits - *And the Freedom Within Them*

Holistic tools are powerful, but they are not panaceas. You cannot meditate away a biochemical condition. You cannot journal your way out of suicidal thoughts. You cannot run five miles and expect your brain to ignore a sudden, severe drop in estrogen. It doesn't work like that.

And yet. These tools still matter.

They matter because they offer you *agency*. They matter because they are often *accessible*. They matter because they honour the whole of you, not just your symptoms, but your soul.

They are not replacements for medical care. But they can sit alongside it, helping you build a life that is a little softer, a little steadier, a little more your own.

You are not failing if therapy doesn't "fix" it. You are not failing if you eat crisps at midnight. You are not failing if you cannot bring yourself to move. These are tools, not tests. And your value is not defined by how well you use them.

Building a Toolkit, Not a To-Do List

PMDD is not a lifestyle problem. It is not a wellness gap. It is a complex, systemic condition that requires proper medical care. But your body is still worth tending. Your mind is still worth soothing. Your nervous system is still worth regulating. Not to fix the condition, but to hold you through it.

Think of these holistic practices not as cures, but as companions. They walk beside you. They remind you that you are not powerless. They offer small kindnesses in the face of something massive.

You deserve every tool available. Medical. Holistic. Emotional. Practical. You deserve a whole toolbox, and the freedom to use what works for *you*.

You do not have to choose between therapy and medication. Between yoga and SSRIs. Between nutrition and hormone treatment. You can build a multi-layered support system that meets you where you are, and holds space for where you're going.

That is what real healing looks like. Not perfection. Not elimination. But support. Integration. Care.

9.3 Building a Personal Protocol

Trial, Error, and Adapting What Works

There comes a point, after the diagnosis, after the chaos, after the crash, when you sit down and ask yourself a question that sounds simple but is actually quite radical: *What do I need to survive this?*

Not what works for everyone else. Not what you're supposed to do. Not what Instagram wellness accounts suggest. But *you*. Your body. Your life. Your cycle. Your mind.

PMDD doesn't respond to a one-size-fits-all treatment plan. It isn't the kind of condition where a doctor hands you a prescription, you take it, and everything slots into place. For most, the journey forward is not linear. It is not tidy. It is frustrating. But it is also deeply personal. And it can be empowering.

Building your own protocol is about turning survival into strategy. It means paying attention to your patterns. It means experimenting with different tools. It means learning what helps and what hurts. It is, by nature, imperfect. You won't always get it right. But you will get better at listening to yourself. And that, in itself, is progress.

Some people start with medication. Others with diet. Others with journaling or movement or therapy. Some are thrown into the deep end after a mental health crisis and have to scramble to piece together support after the fact. There is no wrong place to begin. What matters is that you begin at all.

It helps to think of your protocol as a working document. It is not something etched in stone. It is not something that stays the same forever. It shifts with your cycle, your life stage, your hormone levels, your stress, your access to care. The more flexible you allow it to be, the more sustainable it becomes.

You may find that SSRIs take the edge off your most intense mood swings, but leave you feeling flat. You may try switching to luteal-phase dosing and notice a little more energy return. You might try a different medication and find it works better for sleep but makes your stomach unsettled. These aren't failures. They are data points.

The same goes for lifestyle supports. Maybe yoga helps some months and irritates you others. Maybe journaling helps in the follicular phase, but in the luteal phase, it just brings your spiralling thoughts into sharper focus. Maybe eating more regularly stabilises your mood, but only if you're also getting enough sleep. Each observation teaches you something about how your body responds to change.

At some point, you may discover that your symptoms are heavily tied to stress. That when work is overwhelming or relationships are strained, PMDD hits harder. This doesn't mean stress *causes* PMDD, but it might amplify it. Your protocol might need to include preventative rest. Not just sleep, but actual recovery. Time away from screens. Time away from expectations. Even if it's just ten minutes of quiet in a locked bathroom.

You might experiment with cycle tracking, and notice you feel more anxious after ovulation. Maybe you start writing down symptoms day by day. Maybe you colour-code your calendar so you can see, at a glance, which days are danger zones. Over time, you might start to spot patterns. Not perfectly, but enough to give you a sense of what's coming. This alone can be a relief. It gives you a chance to prepare. To soften your schedule. To ask for help in advance.

Adapting what works often means accepting that what works *now* may not work later. Hormonal landscapes change. Stress levels fluctuate. What helped in your twenties might not land the same way in your thirties. And that's not regression. That's the reality of a dynamic body. Your protocol has to evolve with you.

There is often grief in this process. Grief that it has to be so hard. Grief that your health has become a project. Grief that you can't just live like other people do. But alongside the grief can come pride. Because building your own system is an act of radical care. It is a refusal to abandon yourself in the face of a condition that often demands you do just that.

You might eventually create your own emergency plan. You may have a set of actions you take when symptoms become too much. Maybe it's a bag by the bed with medication, snacks, and a playlist. Maybe it's a document you share with loved ones that explains what you need and what to avoid. These things don't prevent PMDD from hitting. But they give you a sense of control in the middle of the storm.

And yes, you will forget your own plan sometimes. You will find yourself on the bathroom floor wondering why nothing is working. You will forget what helped last cycle. You will doubt yourself. You will wonder if you're back at square one. But the truth is, you're not. Every month you try again, you are learning. You are recalibrating. You are tuning in.

One of the biggest challenges of PMDD is the way it shatters your sense of consistency. You don't feel like yourself all month. You're in survival mode half the time. Building a protocol doesn't eliminate this. But it offers a way to steady the boat. It gives you rituals, reminders, and resources that say, "You've been here before. You survived it. You can again."

Some people write their protocols down. Others keep them in their heads. Some have them printed and laminated. Some scribble them on sticky notes and shove them in drawers. The format doesn't matter. What matters is that it reflects *you*. That it serves *you*. That it honours what *you* need.

Your protocol might include medications, therapy, and supplements. It might involve strict boundaries around certain weeks of the month. It might include specific foods, people you trust, reminders to cancel plans, or routines that help you feel human. It might change every cycle, or stay the same for years. There is no right way. There is only your way.

And yes, it takes effort. It takes energy. And some months, you won't have any of that to give. That's okay too. You're allowed to have off months. You're allowed to forget your own wisdom. The goal isn't perfection. It's continuity. It's saying, *I will keep coming back to myself, even when it's hard.*

PMDD takes a lot from you. But building your own protocol is a way of taking something back. It's an act of resistance. Of restoration. Of refusing to surrender entirely.

You deserve to be supported. And until that support is widespread and built into systems and healthcare and culture, you have every right to build it yourself.

Not because it should be your responsibility.

PART

Ten

When Nothing Works

10.1 When You've Tried It All

The despair of treatment resistance

There can come a point when the options blur into each other. You sit in front of another specialist, another well-meaning professional with a clipboard or a kind expression, and you brace yourself for the next suggestion. You already know what it will be. You've heard it before. Maybe it's an antidepressant, or a new type of birth control, or a referral to someone who "might be able to help." Each time, you nod. You take the leaflet. You try, because what else is there?

But what happens when nothing works? Not just once. Not just a single failed trial or a bad reaction. But a string of hopeful starts that unravel into side effects, spirals, or simply no change at all. When you've read every forum, followed every recommendation, adjusted your diet, cut out caffeine, added yoga, tried magnesium, cried on the floor, begged for answers, and still… the storm returns.

This is the brutal reality of treatment-resistant PMDD. It's not just frustrating. It is soul-shaking. You start to wonder if you're broken in a way that can't be fixed. Not hormonal. Not mental. Not even physical anymore. Just a kind of cursed wiring that defies explanation. And worst of all, it keeps happening on a schedule. You can't even pretend it's random. The same sabotage, month after month.

The word resistance makes it sound clinical. Like something that can be measured, tracked, categorized. But for the person living it, resistance feels like a slow erosion of hope. You try a medication, it fails. You tweak your lifestyle, it fails. You put your faith in one more protocol, one more supplement, one more doctor. Fail. Fail. Fail. You start to fear the very act of trying.

And yet, you do. Because not trying is scarier. Because the pain of living like this is worse than the side effects, the exhaustion, the cost. You become your own experiment. You study your body like it's a hostile terrain. You journal, chart, track symptoms, compare notes, eliminate triggers. You cross-reference articles at 2 a.m., watching videos about neurotransmitters, gut health, trauma recovery, and hormonal cascades. You whisper to yourself that if you just *understand it better*, maybe you'll finally unlock the path out.

People tell you to be patient. Healing takes time. Bodies are complicated. But the problem with PMDD is that it doesn't wait. It doesn't take a break while you explore options or slowly ease into a new plan. It punches through, month after month, with a predictability that feels like a sentence. You don't get recovery time. You don't get to pause the destruction.

What happens to a person when they've tried it all? They often become invisible. The healthcare system doesn't quite know what to do with someone who doesn't respond. You might be offered more aggressive measures, or sometimes less. Sometimes you're just gently dropped. You've tried everything, so maybe the problem is how you're perceiving it. Maybe you're just sensitive. Or noncompliant. Or catastrophizing. You start to internalize those words.

And beneath the exhaustion, there is rage. Not just at the condition, but at the silence around this level of suffering. Rage at the idea that your life is being shredded by something so misunderstood, so underfunded, so frequently dismissed. There are days you wonder if you're exaggerating. Then you remember the hospital visits, the self-harm scars, the medications stacked in the cupboard, the nights curled on the bathroom floor trying to stop yourself from making a permanent decision in a temporary state.

You don't want pity. You want options. You want science that is caught up with your reality. You want treatments that acknowledge this isn't just "PMS turned up a bit," but something far more complex. You want clinicians who have heard of PMDD before you say the acronym. You want a research paper that describes your experience and offers something besides a shrug at the end.

The hardest part is explaining this despair to others. Even to people who love you. You say, "I've tried everything," and they ask, "Have you tried walking more?" Or "What about cutting out sugar?" You want to scream. But you don't. You nod, smile, and try not to cry. You don't want to scare them. You don't want to be a burden.

And then there's grief. Grief for the years lost to trying. Grief for the money spent, the side effects endured, the relationships strained, the jobs lost, the potential unrealized. You can look back at your twenties or thirties and see a patchwork of damage. Not because you didn't try hard enough, but because you tried *too hard*. You gave your body to medicine. You gave your time to healing. You gave your soul to every scrap of hope that was offered, and now you are tired in a way that rest can't reach.

But here's the truth that no one says loudly enough. Treatment resistance doesn't mean you are beyond help. It means the tools available have failed you, not the other way around. It means our current understanding of PMDD is incomplete, and you are standing at the edge of that gap. That takes courage. That takes a level of strength that few people will ever understand.

You are not making this up. You are not weak. You are not failing. You are living through something that should never have been this hard to survive. And you're still here. Maybe bloodied. Maybe doubting. Maybe clinging to the last thread of belief. But here.

Some people keep fighting by trying the next thing. Some people survive by stepping back and saying "enough for now." Some advocate. Some retreat. Some do both in the same week. There is no one way to move through the devastation of treatment resistance. But whatever your path looks like, it deserves respect.

If you are in this place, the place of having tried it all and finding nothing that sticks, please know this book sees you. This chapter is yours. Not because we have a miracle solution, but because we believe your suffering is real, and your story is worth telling. There are researchers out there who haven't given up. There are fellow fugitives who are sharing data, writing letters, marching, and building the future you deserve.

10.2 Hard Decisions

Hysterectomy, menopause, and radical interventions

There is a moment, sometimes after years of fighting, when your mind drifts to the most extreme option. Not out of desperation, but clarity. A deep, almost primal knowing that something inside is waging war on you and the only way to end it might be to take it out. For some, this moment comes quietly. For others, it roars in after yet another failed treatment, another breakdown, another week stolen by rage, terror, or numbness. The thought enters: what if I just got rid of the whole system?

Hysterectomy. That word carries weight. It carries stories of loss and relief, grief and power. It is not just a medical procedure. It is the decision to take control of something that has never felt under your control. For many with PMDD, hysterectomy is not about fertility, not about motherhood, not about a quick fix. It is about survival.

To even consider it is an emotional reckoning. You weigh your pain against your future. You measure the quality of your life against the risks. You run scenarios in your head on repeat. What if it works? What if it doesn't? What if I never feel this way again? What if I wake up and I've lost something that can't be regained?

Some people are told they are too young. Some are dismissed entirely. "That's a drastic step," the doctors say. As if you haven't already taken drastic steps just to stay alive. They want you to be sure. To tick every box. To prove you're not being dramatic. So you wait. You try more medications. You track more symptoms. You suffer longer. All to be taken seriously.

Then there's the issue of what type of hysterectomy. Leaving the ovaries means the hormonal cycle continues, and for PMDD, the issue is not the uterus. It's the hormonal fluctuations driven by the ovaries. So to really silence the storm, an oophorectomy is often needed. The removal of the ovaries. Which means menopause. Instantly.

That opens a whole new set of fears. You are not just trading one struggle for another. You are stepping into a chapter most people don't expect to face until their fifties or sixties. And you are doing it on purpose. Surgical menopause is not gentle. There is no gradual decline. It is sudden, and sometimes brutal. Hot flushes, night sweats, bone density concerns, libido changes, mood swings. You don't know if what's coming will be better or just differently hard.

You start researching hormone replacement therapy. You join forums where others have done it and speak with raw honesty. Some say it saved them. Some say it helped a little. Some are still struggling. There is no guarantee. No certainty. Only the quiet conviction that the way things are now cannot continue.

People might not understand. They might ask why you would do something so final. You try to explain that it is not about being dramatic. It is about being realistic. You have watched your life shrink around this condition. You have lost days, weeks, entire months. Relationships have suffered. Careers have stalled. Joy has dulled. You have already lost so much. You are simply drawing a line.

There is also grief. Grief for a body that has failed you. Grief for the children you may have wanted. Even if you never planned to have children, the decision to remove that possibility can still sting. It is a mourning of what might have been. And it is okay to feel that. You can grieve and still be certain.

And then, there is hope. A quiet, trembling kind of hope. That this might actually work. That you might be able to live a life without monthly destruction. That you might stop fearing your own brain. That you might have space to rebuild the pieces of yourself you tucked away in survival mode.

It is a hard decision. It is not one anyone makes lightly. It demands bravery, resilience, and the kind of strength that few people ever have to call on. But if you are here, standing at that edge, it means you are thinking clearly. It means you are listening to yourself. It means you are refusing to settle for a life ruled by suffering.

No one can make the choice for you. Not a doctor, not a partner, not a parent. This is your body, your future, your pain. And whatever you decide, that decision deserves to be respected. Whether you pursue surgery or not. Whether you wait or move forward. Whether you change your mind later.

Some people find peace after surgery. Some find improvement with hormone therapy. Some find that it opens a new chapter that is not perfect, but finally liveable. Some don't find full relief, but still feel the decision gave them back a sense of agency. That, in itself, can be life changing.

10.3 Crisis Planning & Harm Reduction
Managing the unmanageable

There are days, sometimes whole weeks, when PMDD feels completely unmanageable. Not difficult. Not distressing. But like a tidal wave crashing through your life with no warning and no escape. These are the moments when your thoughts scare you. When the darkness feels so total that it's hard to believe it will ever lift. When your body feels like a stranger and your mind feels like an enemy. These are the crisis points. And they are not just dramatic moments in a story. They are real. They are dangerous. They are survivable. But they must be taken seriously.

For some, the first crisis comes out of nowhere. You're having what seems like a normal day, and then the spiral starts. A thought becomes a conviction. A mistake becomes a symbol. A memory becomes an accusation. You feel everything all at once, and nothing at all. You might cry without knowing why. You might feel like your body is on fire or like you've gone completely numb. You might have the thought that you do not want to be alive. And it doesn't come gently. It arrives fully formed. Not because you want to die, but because you want the pain to stop.

These moments are terrifying. And often, they come with shame. You think, why can't I control this? Why can't I just hold on a little better? Why am I thinking this again when I was doing so well last week? But PMDD is not a matter of willpower. It is not something you can think your way out of when the chemistry of your brain is working against you.

This is where crisis planning matters. Not as a cure. Not as a way to avoid all risk. But as a way to give yourself a rope to hold onto when the current gets too strong. It's not about fixing the storm. It's about building a raft.

A crisis plan can be simple. It can be a note in your phone. A printed sheet taped to your bathroom mirror. A message you pre-write and save for when your words disappear. It can be a list of who to contact, where to go, what to say. It can include reminders of what you have survived before. Photos of the people or places you want to return to. It can be a phrase that keeps you tethered. Even just one: hold on.

Some people find it helpful to write a letter to their future self. Something you create when you are in your clear mind. Something that says, I know this pain will come again. But I also know it ends. I have seen it end. Please just hold on. You do not have to believe it when you read it. You only have to read it.

Harm reduction is not about perfection. It is about survival. It is about recognizing that you may not be able to avoid every crash, but you can soften the landing. You can remove sharp objects. You can delay decisions. You can make a plan with someone you trust. You can agree that during your worst days, you will not be alone. You can choose to do the minimum, not the maximum. You can stay alive, even if you don't feel like living.

There is nothing weak about needing help. There is nothing shameful about planning for the worst. It means you understand your condition. It means you are taking it seriously. It means you want to live. Even when you don't feel that want in the moment. Even when your brain lies to you and says you are a burden or a failure or beyond saving. Having a plan in place is an act of resistance against that lie.

Sometimes, harm reduction looks like going to bed early just to escape the evening spiral. Sometimes it's watching the same movie three nights in a row because it keeps your mind anchored. Sometimes it's eating whatever you can, not what you're "supposed" to. Sometimes it's choosing not to respond to messages because conserving energy is more important than politeness. These are not failures. They are strategies. And they are valid.

You might not be able to eliminate every dangerous thought. But you can learn to recognize when you are slipping. You can practice reaching out before it gets too deep. You can talk about what a crisis looks like for you with the people who care about you. You can teach them how to spot the signs and what to do if you start to disappear.

For some, crisis planning includes keeping emergency medication on hand. For others, it's a direct line to a therapist or a crisis text service. For many, it is a community of people who understand PMDD and can hold space for the mess, not just the recovery. These things do not fix the illness. But they make it possible to survive the worst of it.

If you are reading this and have never made a crisis plan, let this be your invitation. Not because you are weak, but because you are brave enough to admit that some days will be too hard to face alone. If you have made one, revisit it. Update it. Share it with someone who can hold it for you. If you've needed it recently, you are not broken. You are human, living through something very few people truly understand.

There is a version of you that exists beyond this chapter. You do not have to believe that today. Just keep walking toward it. Even if that walk is slow. Even if you crawl.

Managing the unmanageable doesn't mean controlling it. It means knowing it's coming and preparing to survive it. That is not giving up. That is staying. That is enduring. That is living through the fire instead of becoming it.

.

PART

Eleven

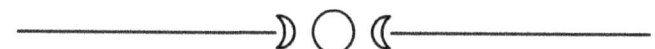

Surviving the Luteal Phase

11.1 When You Feel the Shift

Early Warning Signs and Preparation

It starts in a silence I almost miss,
a thought that bites where it used to kiss.
The air gets heavier, my skin too tight,
a shadow moves in, swallowing light.

I blink, and I'm gone, replaced by a scream,
a woman unravelled, caught in a dream.
The mirror holds someone I don't survive,
and still, somehow, I'm breathing, alive.

No siren, no warning, just the crash,
a mind in flames, a system rash.
One body, two selves, torn at the seam.
I mourn who I was like a half-lost dream.

There is a moment, often quiet but unmistakable, when the shift happens. It might be so subtle you nearly talk yourself out of believing it's real. A pang of irritability that feels too sharp for the situation. A flicker of self-doubt that moves in like a cloud. The world hasn't changed, but something inside you has. You know it. Even if you don't want to. The luteal phase is coming, and with it, the slide into symptoms that can hijack your entire self.

Recognizing this shift early is one of the most powerful tools you can develop. You may not be able to stop what's coming, but you can brace for it. You can prepare your mind, body, and life in small, intentional ways that soften the blow. It starts with learning to hear your own alarm bells before they start screaming.

For some, the warning signs arrive like clockwork: sleep disturbances, bloating, skin changes, a sudden drop in mood, or intense hunger. For others, it's more emotional. An inexplicable sense of dread. Thoughts that spiral faster than usual. The way music suddenly sounds too loud or how social plans feel like a threat instead of a joy. You might find yourself picking fights or crying at a commercial. These early changes are not imaginary. They're your body signalling a neurological and hormonal shift that can't be seen but can absolutely be felt.

One of the most helpful steps is to keep track of your cycle—not just the dates but the symptoms. Write down what happens in the days leading up to your luteal phase. Keep a journal, use an app, or simply note it in your calendar. This practice doesn't just give you data, it gives you validation. When you can look back and say, yes, this happened last month too, and the month before that, it becomes harder to gaslight yourself. You stop feeling like a failure for falling apart and start seeing a pattern. A pattern that you didn't cause but can begin to plan for.

Once you know your red flags, the next step is to build a gentle response plan. Think of it like preparing for a storm. You check the forecast, gather supplies, and secure the windows—not because you can change the weather, but because you can reduce the damage.

Maybe your first move is simplifying your schedule. If you're someone who tends to take on too much, this is the time to decline extra commitments. Push back non-urgent appointments. Let people know you might be slower to reply. You don't have to explain everything, but you can quietly create space.

Another important tactic is prepping your environment. Small changes can make a big difference when you're in survival mode. Stock the fridge with easy, nourishing foods. Lay out soft clothes that don't trigger sensory overwhelm. If noise is an issue, charge your noise-cancelling headphones. If sleep becomes difficult, prepare a wind-down routine now while you still have the energy to do it. You're building a nest that can hold you when everything else feels unsteady.

It's also helpful to make a short, practical list of coping strategies, things that genuinely help you, not just the things you think should. Maybe it's taking a warm bath, watching a show that comforts you, going for a slow walk, or texting a friend who won't try to fix you. Maybe it's cancelling everything and crawling under a weighted blanket. You don't need to be productive. You need to be kind. You need a version of yourself that understands this is not the time for pushing through, but for softening in.

Emotionally, it helps to name what's happening. Say it out loud. Write it down. "I feel the shift." This isn't weakness. It's awareness. Acknowledging the change gives you a moment of separation from it. You are not the storm. You are the person who felt the first drop of rain and went inside for shelter. This self-awareness is a form of power. It's the beginning of choice.

There will be days when even preparation feels futile. When symptoms crash in harder than expected. When the strategies that once worked seem flimsy. On those days, the goal is not perfection. It's preservation. Try to hold on to the idea that this is temporary. The version of you who is falling apart is not the whole story. She is in distress, not in truth. When you start to believe her thoughts, pause. If you can't talk back to them yet, write them down. Set them aside. Promise to revisit them in ten days. Not everything the luteal phase says is a lie, but it rarely speaks with balance.

You might also consider writing a note to yourself when you're in a better place. A letter from your follicular self to your luteal self. It can be simple. Just a reminder that this has happened before and passed. That your brain is inflamed, not broken. That even when it feels like the world is crumbling, your worth hasn't changed. You can tuck this note into a drawer, or keep it in your phone. It's your message in a bottle to the future you who might forget what calm feels like.

Support systems can also be part of your early response plan. Let someone you trust know where you are in your cycle. You don't have to go into detail. You can say something like, "I'm heading into my tough week—just giving you a heads-up." That small moment of connection can reduce shame and create accountability. It also gives others a chance to show up for you in small but meaningful ways.

When you live with PMDD, the luteal phase becomes a battleground. But learning to spot the shift is like noticing the rustle in the leaves before the wind picks up. It won't stop the storm, but it gives you a chance to hold on to something before it hits. Over time, this awareness becomes its own form of resilience. Not because you become invincible, but because you learn to meet yourself where you are. With preparation. With softness. With the quiet knowledge that you are doing your best to survive something invisible, unpredictable, and immensely real.

11.2 Luteal Survival Kit

What to Pack Emotionally, Physically, Socially

When you're dealing with PMDD, surviving the luteal phase can feel like being dropped into the middle of a storm with no warning, no shelter, and no supplies. That's why preparing your own survival kit is not just a nice idea, it's essential. This isn't about stocking up on optimism or pretending it's not that bad. This is about arming yourself with real, useful tools that support you in every area of your life during the hardest days.

Start with your physical needs. Your body is on the front line, reacting to hormonal chaos that can leave you aching, bloated, exhausted, and overstimulated. Your kit might include items that soothe and comfort. Think of clothes that feel soft and non-restrictive, things that won't make you want to scream just from touching your skin. Keep a stash of heat packs for cramps or back pain, magnesium if it helps you, and snacks that are easy to digest but still grounding. If food becomes difficult, focus on simple choices that offer steady energy without adding guilt. Stocking your kitchen with the right things beforehand means one less decision when your brain is full of static.

Sleep can become elusive during the luteal phase. You may struggle to fall asleep, wake often, or experience strange, intense dreams that leave you more tired than before. Prepare a sleep space that invites calm. That might mean blackout curtains, earplugs, a white noise machine, or a calming scent like lavender. If your thoughts tend to spiral at night, consider keeping a notebook beside your bed just to offload your brain before you close your eyes. Even if sleep doesn't come easily, rest still matters. Give yourself permission to lie still without judgment. Even moments of stillness count.

Next, think about your emotional needs. This is often where the pain hits hardest. You may feel hopeless, irritable, confused, overwhelmed, ashamed, or detached. It's not always possible to stop those feelings, but it is possible to meet them with support instead of silence. One powerful tool is a letter or message written by your stable self. Keep it somewhere you can reach easily. It might remind you that what you're feeling is cyclical, not permanent. That your thoughts are being filtered through the lens of a biochemical storm. That the voice in your head right now is not the only truth. Even a short message like "This will pass. You've been here before. You will come out again" can act like an anchor.

Make space in your kit for emotional comfort items. They may seem small, but they serve as touchstones when everything feels slippery. A favourite jumper. A playlist that makes you feel less alone. A TV show that distracts without overstimulating. A worn book you've read a hundred times. These things don't need to be impressive. They need to be familiar. PMDD often makes the world feel alien and threatening. Repetition and softness are grounding forces.

Your social world also needs attention. PMDD has a way of isolating people. You may find yourself snapping at loved ones, withdrawing from friends, or feeling convinced that no one could possibly understand what you're going through. That's why your kit should include social lifelines. Choose one or two people you trust. Let them know what PMDD looks like for you. You don't need to bare your soul every time. A simple message like "I'm in it right now" can be enough to open a door. If you can, create a code or shorthand with them so you don't have to explain everything when you're already depleted.

Not every social need involves reaching out. Sometimes, the survival tactic is creating boundaries. Your kit should include permission to cancel, to say no, to protect your energy. It helps to pre-prepare a few kind, clear messages for when you need space. You can write them in advance and send them when needed, so you're not scrambling for words while overwhelmed. Examples might be, "I care about you, but I need some time to myself this week," or, "I'm going quiet for a bit. I'll reach out when I can."

You might also consider building a tiny ritual into your day that reminds you you're not disappearing. Something that connects you back to yourself, even if it's only for a few minutes. Maybe it's lighting a candle in the morning, scribbling one sentence in a journal, stretching your arms to the ceiling when you wake up. These are signals to your nervous system that you are still here. Still tethered. Still human in the midst of something that tries to unravel you.

Technology can be a tool or a trigger. If you know that certain apps make you feel worse, uninstall them for this part of your cycle. If social media fuels comparison or agitation, give yourself permission to step away. Replace that scroll time with something that nurtures you. A nature documentary. A guided meditation. A photo album. A puzzle game that doesn't require emotional investment. Curate your digital world to match your capacity.

Include reminders that this isn't your fault. You didn't choose this. You aren't weak because you need extra help right now. You are responding to a legitimate, biological condition. Survival isn't about getting through it all with a smile. It's about figuring out what makes you feel even one percent more safe, one percent more okay, and making space for that thing.

A luteal survival kit is not a miracle cure. It won't take the pain away. But it will soften the impact. It will remind you that you are not powerless. You are not broken. You are someone who has learned to anticipate the tide and prepare her ground. That is not weakness. That is strategy. That is care. That is strength disguised as softness.

And when the cycle ends and you begin to return to yourself, take time to look back and reflect. Did something help more than expected? Was there something missing that you needed? Use that knowledge to adjust your kit for next time. Each cycle is another chance to understand yourself better. Not to fix yourself, but to care for yourself more completely.

Because surviving PMDD is not about waiting to be rescued. It's about building the raft with whatever materials you have, holding on tight, and reminding yourself, this storm does pass. And when it comes again, you'll be ready.

11.3 Scripts for Support

How to Ask for Help (Even When It's Hard)

Asking for help when you're drowning feels counterintuitive. PMDD can wrap your brain in a blanket of shame, isolation, and fear. You might think you'll sound dramatic. Or needy. Or that no one will understand anyway. But here's the truth: you are allowed to need help. Especially when your hormones have hijacked your nervous system and you're fighting just to stay afloat.

The hardest part is often knowing what to say. Even people who love you can't read your mind. In the depths of the luteal phase, words can disappear, or come out all wrong. That's why having simple, pre-thought-out scripts can be a lifeline. They take the pressure off when you have nothing left. You don't have to explain your whole life story. You just need a way to open the door.

Start with the smallest version of help. Sometimes what you need isn't a full rescue but just for someone to know you're struggling. You can try saying something like, "I'm in a rough patch right now. Just letting you know I might be a bit quiet." This doesn't ask anything from the other person, but it signals your internal weather. You're making space for honesty without placing a burden.

If you do need something more tangible, being specific is key. Vague cries for help often go unanswered not because people don't care, but because they genuinely don't know what to do. Try narrowing it down. You could say, "Could you pick up something from the shop for me?" or "Would you be able to sit with me for a bit? I don't need to talk, just not be alone." These kinds of requests can feel awkward to make, but they allow others to show up in practical ways.

It's okay to admit that things feel big. One of the most honest things you can say is, "I'm not doing great. I don't need you to fix it, but I just need someone to know." That sentence can be a bridge out of your own head. When the symptoms of PMDD are raging, you may feel like you're falling apart in secret. Naming your distress out loud, even gently, can bring relief.

If you're afraid people won't understand, you can try explaining it in terms that make sense to them. For example, "This is the part of my cycle where things get really hard. It happens every month. I know it's hormonal, but it still feels real." You're not asking for medical advice. You're asking for space and support. You can follow up with something like, "If I seem different this week, that's why. I'd really appreciate some patience."

For partners, family, or close friends, it helps to have one deeper conversation during your follicular phase, the time when you feel more stable. This is your window to educate, to set expectations, and to ask for backup before the crisis hits. You might say, "There's a pattern in my cycle where I get really low and anxious. It's called PMDD. It's hard for me to communicate when I'm in it, so I'm asking now for support during that time." You can then suggest what kind of support you need. Maybe that's a reminder to eat. Maybe it's a gentle check-in. Maybe it's simply not taking your silence personally.

Even workplaces can benefit from a low-pressure script. You don't have to disclose everything. You might say, "I have a recurring health condition that can flare up for a few days each month. If I seem quieter or need to shift deadlines slightly, that's why. I'm doing my best to manage it proactively." You are not asking for pity. You are communicating a boundary with professionalism.

It's also completely fair to prepare a script for emergencies. Something you can copy, paste, or send in moments of serious distress. You might write one ahead of time that says, "I'm not okay. I don't know what I need, but I know I need someone to check in on me. Please don't ignore this." Save it in your notes app. Keep it somewhere visible. When the time comes, use it. If your brain is telling you not to bother anyone, that you're being a burden, that you'll feel different tomorrow, remember that this is PMDD speaking. This is not your rational self.

Sometimes, people won't respond how you hoped. They may misunderstand. They may dismiss or distance themselves. That hurts. But it doesn't mean you were wrong to ask. Keep trying. Keep reaching for the people who make you feel seen and safe. And if you don't have those people yet, there are communities online who do understand. People who have walked through the same fire. Forums, support groups, helplines. It's not the same as someone sitting beside you in person, but it still counts. That digital connection can be a hand on your shoulder when you're about to fall.

Practice helps too. Try saying the words out loud when you're not in crisis. Let them sit in your mouth. Try them on. The more you practice, the easier it becomes to say them when it matters. Asking for help is a skill. It doesn't mean you're broken. It means you're aware. You know your limits. You're choosing to connect instead of disappearing.

You do not have to suffer in silence to prove you are strong. Strength is knowing when to ask for a hand. When to let someone else carry a little of the weight. When to say, "I need you," even if your voice shakes. Especially then.

PMDD isolates. Asking for help reconnects. And every time you do it, you're not just surviving, you're building a bridge back to yourself.

PART

Twelve

Love in the Luteal Phase

12.1 PMDD and Romance
Explaining, Surviving, and Supporting

Romantic relationships are hard enough.

They require trust, communication, patience, and a willingness to grow alongside another flawed human.

Now throw PMDD into the mix, and suddenly, the terrain shifts. You're not just navigating the ordinary ups and downs of love anymore. You're driving through a storm that appears without warning and sometimes tears everything apart on its way in and out.

When you have PMDD, explaining it to someone you love can feel like trying to describe a dream you keep having, one that changes shape each time you try to pin it down. It's not just a bad mood or some irritability before your period. It's a full-body possession. A shift in personality. A fracture in the connection between who you are and how you behave. It's hard enough to understand it yourself. Asking someone else to understand can feel almost impossible.

The first hurdle is language. How do you explain to a partner that every month, like clockwork, you become someone else? Not in a cute or quirky way. In a way that's frightening. Maybe you rage. Maybe you shut down. Maybe you cry in a way that scares even you. You might accuse them of things they never did or retreat into silence so total it feels like abandonment. You might pick fights you don't mean, say things you would never say in the light of your follicular phase. And then, as quickly as the storm arrived, it lifts. You return to yourself, shocked and ashamed, looking at the damage and wondering how on earth anyone could love you through it.

But some people do. Some people try. Some people want to.

The second hurdle is survival. Once the conversation has been had, once you've named the monster and let your partner peek behind the curtain, you're left with the question: now what? Love doesn't fix PMDD. Neither does compassion, though it softens the edges. Relationships must be built to survive it. They must flex and breathe with it. They must have room for rupture and repair.

Surviving PMDD in a relationship takes structure. That might mean having a shared calendar where your partner knows roughly when the luteal phase begins, so they can prepare too. It might mean agreeing on ways to communicate during that time. Maybe you text instead of talk. Maybe you create a "safe word" that signals you need space, or that a conversation needs to stop before it spirals. Maybe you write each other letters during your follicular days that you can both re-read when things get hard, to remember what is true beneath the chaos.

It also takes realism. There will be moments that are not okay. Words said that leave marks. Confusion. Exhaustion. Your partner may at times feel helpless, or even frightened. It doesn't mean they don't love you. It means they are human. And you are too. Expecting yourself to be a perfect partner while navigating PMDD is cruel. Expecting your partner to be perfectly understanding is also a trap. What you both need is a foundation of honesty and forgiveness, built up over time.

The third piece is support. Not just you being supported, but also supporting your partner as they walk beside you through this. Sometimes the person with PMDD becomes the sole focus, and understandably so, given the intensity of symptoms. But your partner is also living through it. They are impacted by the shifts. They are affected by the silences, the arguments, the unpredictability. And if you want your relationship to survive, their wellbeing matters too.

Support might mean checking in with them after the luteal storm has passed and asking, how was that for you? What did you need that you didn't get? What hurt? What helped? It might mean inviting them to come with you to an appointment, or encouraging them to talk to someone about their experience. You are a team, and sometimes that team needs more than love. It needs tools, education, space, and reinforcements.

Some couples find rituals that help. One woman describes how she and her partner have a "reunion dinner" once her period starts, marking her return to herself. They eat their favourite food, watch a comforting movie, and let themselves feel the relief together. Another couple uses a shared journal to write notes to each other when talking feels too hard. One woman writes, "Even when I hated him in the moment, it helped to see his words the next day. It reminded me that the love hadn't gone anywhere. Just me."

Romance is so often built on the fantasy of ease. That love should be natural, smooth, uncomplicated. PMDD blows a hole through that fantasy. But it doesn't mean love is impossible. In fact, many couples who weather this find that their relationship becomes something stronger, more intimate, more deeply forged by fire. A kind of battle bond. Not a perfect love, but a real one.

And then there's sex and intimacy. The part nobody wants to talk about, but everyone feels. PMDD can make physical touch intolerable. Or desperately craved, but impossible to receive without tears or tension. Desire can vanish. Or become tangled in shame and rage. Some partners take it personally. Others shut down completely. The key here is communication. Not in the moment, necessarily, but in the quiet days. Talk about what feels good, what feels off-limits, what changes when the luteal shift begins. Remind each other that this is a tide, not a verdict. That closeness can look different in different phases.

Romantic love under the weight of PMDD is not a fairytale. It's not linear. It is clumsy and flawed and full of contradiction. You may push someone away and still want them to stay. You may need solitude while craving closeness. You may say things you don't mean, and then weep because you meant the opposite. This is the shape of love when the brain betrays you once a month.

But if someone sees you, truly sees you, even through the storm, that is not something to take lightly. And if you can learn to let yourself be loved, not just when you're at your best but when you're at your most undone, that is its own kind of victory.

PMDD doesn't make you unlovable. It makes you human in a particular, difficult way. But with understanding, with effort, and with grace on both sides, romance can live here. It won't look like the movies. It might be messier, more awkward, and less photogenic. But it will be real. And real love, the kind that survives storms, is the kind that can hold you even when you can't hold yourself.

12.2 Parenting with PMDD

Guilt, Exhaustion, and Presence

There's a horrid ache in being both the safe place and the danger zone, a parent trying to hold steady while the ground keeps giving way. It's not the ordinary exhaustion of raising a child, although that alone can be immense. It's the gut-punch of knowing that the hardest parts of you sometimes show up right when your child needs the softest. It's loving them so deeply and still feeling like you're failing them, not because you don't care, but because something in your brain is warring against your ability to connect, stay calm, or even function.

Parenting is already a relentless act of showing up. With PMDD, that act becomes a monthly tightrope. There are days you can barely speak kindly to yourself, let alone to a small, needy human. There are days when your nerves are so raw that even the sound of their voice can feel like too much. And then the guilt follows, thick and immediate. Not just guilt for snapping or shutting down, but guilt for the look in their eyes when they sense something is wrong and they don't know why.

There are moments when you hide in the bathroom just to breathe. When you turn on the TV not because it's screen time, but because you need silence. When you say, "Not now," to a question that deserves an answer. And all the while, a voice in your head is whispering, "You're not doing this right." That voice is cruel. It doesn't account for the fact that you're doing the best you can with a brain that flips itself inside out once a month.

PMDD doesn't just bring emotional storms. It also brings bone-deep exhaustion. The kind that settles in your limbs and won't lift, even with sleep. Parenting with this kind of tiredness feels like dragging yourself through wet cement. You know what your child needs. You know what they deserve. But the gap between knowing and delivering can feel impossibly wide. You may find yourself doing the bare minimum just to survive. Feeding them, dressing them, making it through the day. And then, when they finally sleep, the guilt crashes in. You replay every sharp word. Every missed opportunity. Every moment you weren't quite present.

But here is what needs to be said: survival is not failure. If you got through the day and your child is safe and fed and knows, even in some small way, that they are loved, that is not nothing. That is everything. Presence is not always about being joyful or energetic. Sometimes it is simply being there, even while falling apart.

Children are intuitive. They can feel when something is off. But they are also resilient. What matters most is not being perfect. What matters is being honest, being consistent in your love, and coming back when you've had to step away. Repair matters more than perfection. If you've lost your temper or shut them out, you can return. You can kneel down and say, "I'm sorry. That wasn't your fault. I'm having a hard time right now, but I love you more than anything." Those words matter more than any flawless performance.

Some parents worry about damaging their children by exposing them to PMDD. That fear is valid. No one wants their child to see them in pain. But shielding them completely is not always possible. What *is* possible is helping them understand. Age-appropriate honesty goes a long way. You can say, "Mummy feels a bit stormy today," or "Sometimes I get really tired and sad before my period. It doesn't mean I don't love you. It just means I need a bit more rest and quiet."

In fact, many children raised by parents with PMDD grow up with a deep empathy and emotional intelligence. They understand that feelings come in waves. That people can struggle and still be safe. That love can exist even inside difficulty. If you model gentleness with yourself, they learn to be gentle with themselves too.

Still, none of this makes it easy. There may be weeks when you feel like you're holding on by a thread. When bedtime feels like a mountain. When play feels impossible. You may look around and feel like every other parent is doing it better. But what you don't see are their private battles. Every parent has them. Yours just happens to be shaped by hormones that sabotage your stability. That doesn't make you a bad parent. It makes you a parent with a specific, invisible challenge.

You are allowed to need help. Whether that's calling in support from a friend or partner, lowering expectations for yourself during the luteal days, or creating rituals that help you stay grounded. Maybe it's as simple as prepping a few activities in advance for the days when your brain shuts down. Maybe it's letting go of the idea that you have to be the perfect parent and instead embracing that being good enough is more than enough.

Your child doesn't need a version of you that's always happy or always on. They need a version of you that tries. That returns. That lets them see that it's okay to struggle and okay to rest. They need a parent who models resilience, not performance.

It's okay if there are days when you don't want to parent. That doesn't make you ungrateful. It makes you honest. And honesty can be a bridge back to yourself. You are allowed to say, "This is hard." You are allowed to mourn the ease that others might have. But in that mourning, don't forget to also see your strength. Every day you keep going, every day you stay, even when your body and mind are screaming for escape, is an act of radical love.

There may be moments in the future when your child asks, "Were you okay back then?" And you might say, "Not always. But I always loved you. And I never stopped trying." That is the kind of presence that leaves a mark. Not the absence of flaws, but the presence of effort.

PMDD and parenting is not a neat combination. But it is a real one. Messy, raw, heartbreaking, and beautiful in its own way. You may never feel like you're doing enough. But you are here. You are trying. And that matters more than you know.

12.3 Friendship, Family, and Boundaries
Protecting Your Peace

When you live with PMDD, relationships that once felt effortless can begin to feel sharp around the edges. Even the most well-meaning friend or family member can start to feel like a trigger. Sometimes it's the casual dismissal, the "Everyone gets moody before their period." Sometimes it's the silence when you need to be seen. Sometimes it's the expectation that you keep showing up the way you always have, even when you're crumbling inside.

And then of course there's the weight of it all. Wanting to be the daughter, the sibling, the friend who answers messages on time, who remembers birthdays, who doesn't cancel at the last minute or go quiet for two weeks straight. You may have once been the reliable one, the one who made the effort. Now, during your luteal days, even replying to a text feels like work. Social energy becomes a currency you don't have. And underneath the quietness, there's often guilt. You want to be present. You want to explain. But sometimes there are no words that can do it justice.

Boundaries become necessary. Not in a harsh or dramatic way, but in a quiet, protective one. You start to learn which relationships feed you and which ones drain you. You start to notice who holds space for your experience without trying to fix or minimize it. And you start to recognise that you can still love people and need distance. That both things can be true at once.

Family dynamics can be especially complicated. Maybe they don't believe in PMDD. Maybe they see it as an excuse. Maybe they don't understand why you've changed or why you can't just "snap out of it." Or maybe they mean well but make it worse with endless advice, unsolicited opinions, or comparisons to their own experiences. Trying to explain PMDD to someone who hasn't lived it can feel like shouting underwater. You use all the right words, and still, they don't seem to land.

It's okay to stop trying to convince people who are unwilling to listen. It doesn't mean you've failed. It means you're choosing your peace. You are not responsible for managing other people's comfort at the cost of your own sanity. You are allowed to set limits. You are allowed to say, "I can't talk about this right now," or "That topic is off-limits," or even, "I need space from this relationship."

Friendship, too, can change in the face of PMDD. Some people drift. Some disappear altogether. It hurts, deeply. Especially if they were there in your lighter phases and gone when things got dark. But it also clears space. And sometimes, in that space, new kinds of friendships emerge. The kind built not on constant availability but mutual respect. The kind where you can say, "I'm in my luteal phase," and they get it. No questions, no judgement. Just quiet understanding.

These friendships are gold. They might not be loud or flashy. They might be made up of voice notes, check-ins, or someone dropping off a meal without making you talk. They might not demand explanations. They might not keep score. They simply show up in a way that allows you to be exactly as you are.

If you are lucky enough to have people like that in your life, hold them close. And if you don't yet, know that they exist. Sometimes they come from the most unexpected places. A support group. An online community. A friend of a friend who knows the terrain. Sometimes just one person believing you is enough to shift everything.

You don't have to explain your boundaries to everyone. And you don't have to feel guilty for having them. Saying no is a kindness to yourself. Saying, "I love you, but I need time," is an act of care. You are allowed to prioritise your wellbeing, even if it disappoints others. Discomfort is not the same as harm. And self-protection is not selfishness.

Protecting your peace might mean taking a step back from social plans in your luteal phase. It might mean turning off your phone. It might mean not engaging in conversations that leave you feeling worse. It might even mean letting go of relationships that no longer serve you. There is grief in that. But there is also relief.

Over time, you will start to build a life that holds you. One where you don't feel like you're constantly failing other people. One where your energy isn't spent performing wellness for the comfort of others. One where the people around you don't just tolerate your limits but respect them.

PMDD is already loud. Already overwhelming. The last thing you need is more noise from relationships that take more than they give. Protecting your peace is not a luxury. It's a necessity. It is the ground you build your healing on. It is what allows you to keep going, even on the hardest days.

You are not too much. You are not a burden. You are a human being doing your best inside a body that turns against itself once a month. The people who truly love you will learn how to meet you there. Not always perfectly. But with effort. With compassion. With room for the real you, not just the easy version.

You deserve that. You deserve boundaries. You deserve peace.

PART

Thirteen

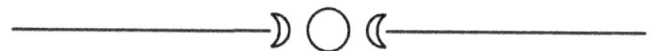

Stories of Survival

Talia, 23

I used to count the days until I lost myself again. One week I was laughing with friends, doing well at school, thinking maybe life was getting easier. Then I'd wake up and it was like something had snapped. I'd cry for hours. Shout at people I loved. Feel like dying. I thought I was dramatic, or weak, or just... broken. My mum thought it was teenage hormones until one day she found me sobbing in the bathtub saying I didn't want to be alive. That's when things changed. A female GP listened, really listened. She said, "This might be PMDD." That name saved me. I track now. I have a plan. I breathe through it. Some days are still hell, but I know it isn't all me. That knowledge? It gave me back my life.

Jess, 26

I was misdiagnosed for five years. Depression. Anxiety. BPD. Nothing ever *fit*. I'd be fine, and then out of nowhere I'd want to burn my life down. Relationships ruined. Jobs quit. One night, in a rabbit hole of desperation, I found a Reddit thread. Someone described what I was feeling, *exactly*, and said the words: "PMDD nearly killed me too." I cried for an hour. From there, I found others. I found treatment. I still struggle, but I'm not alone. I'm not crazy. And every month I survive feels like a tiny revolution.

Lena, 34

My children would look at me like I was a stranger. I'd scream, shut doors, disappear into silence. And then, a few days later, I'd be back, begging for forgiveness, broken with shame. I thought they deserved better. I almost left. Thought they'd be safer without me. It wasn't until a therapist quietly asked about my cycle that I started tracking. The pattern screamed back at me. PMDD. I wept. Not with defeat, but relief. I wasn't a monster. I had a condition. I got support. I started medication. And I made a promise to stay. To survive this, month by month. For them. For me.

Bea, 43

By 43, I'd been dismissed by doctors more times than I could count. Told to meditate. Exercise. "Get more sleep." I was articulate and professional, and still no one believed me when I said I felt like a different person half the month. It took demanding a referral, keeping detailed symptom charts, and breaking down in a consultant's office to finally be heard. I now run a local PMDD support group. We meet monthly, share stories, and cry. It's the most human, healing thing I've ever been part of. I found purpose in the pain.

Lorna, 52

At 52, I was done. Thirty years of this war with myself. I tried
everything. Pills. Therapy. Diets. Holistic nonsense. It stole my
marriage. My career. My joy. My last option? A hysterectomy.
People warned me it was extreme, but I was already living in
extremes. I had nothing left to lose. I did it, and for the first time
since I was a teenager, I felt peace. Real peace. It's not the answer
for everyone. But for me? It was rebirth. I mourned my body's
betrayal. Then I reclaimed it.

6. Elsie, 68

I didn't know the word PMDD existed until I was 65. I thought I'd
just been a bad wife. A moody mother. A difficult woman. The
rages, the spirals, the empty days where I felt nothing at all, I carried
them like shameful secrets. It wasn't until my granddaughter went
through it and sent me an article that I wept with recognition. I
wish I had known. I wish someone had told me it wasn't my fault.
But I tell people now. I talk. I share. I forgive myself. That's what
survival looks like at this age: grace.

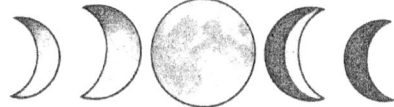

Sometimes slowly, sometimes all at once, the fog lifts. You wake up and feel it in your body first. A lightness. A breath that reaches all the way to the bottom of your lungs. You notice that you're not bracing anymore. The world softens at the edges. You make coffee and it tastes like coffee, not static. Someone asks how you are and you answer without having to lie.

These are the "good days." The days that feel like coming home.

After everything you've survived, even the good days can be hard to trust. Joy doesn't feel safe at first. Peace feels suspicious. You wait for the drop. For the hormones to creep back in and set fire to all the calm. You hesitate to make plans. You hesitate to hope.

That's okay. It makes sense. When you've lived through a war inside your body, peace can feel unfamiliar. But little by little, these good days become more than just breaks in the storm. They become the place you begin to rebuild from.

Rebuilding doesn't mean pretending nothing happened. It doesn't mean erasing the darkness or minimizing your pain. It means creating a life that acknowledges what you've lived through and still makes room for joy. Not perfect joy. Not uninterrupted joy. But real, grounded, earned joy.

It might be as simple as letting yourself laugh again without guilt. Or reaching out to someone you trust, not because you need saving, but because you want connection. It might be trying something new, even if it scares you. Booking the class. Planting the seed. Writing the sentence. Or just sitting still in the rare, sacred quiet of a stable mind.

There is power in learning how to live with PMDD, but there is equal power in learning how to live *beyond* it. Not because it disappears. Not because it gets easier. But because you get wiser. You begin to track your patterns. You learn what to avoid and what to embrace. You recognise the first signs of the shift and act sooner. You develop tools. You soften your inner voice. You give yourself grace.

You become fluent in your own experience.

And in doing so, you begin to rewrite the story. You are no longer just surviving the month. You are authoring your own rhythm. Maybe that rhythm includes rest before you need it. Maybe it includes asking for help without shame. Maybe it means saying no more often. Maybe it means saying yes to things you once thought you'd lost the right to want.

You start to move through your life not as someone who is broken, but as someone who is living with complexity. There is dignity in that. There is resilience in it. There is even beauty in it.

The "good days" aren't just a break from suffering. They are a vital part of the story. They remind you who you are beneath the biochemical chaos. They remind you of what's still possible. They help you recover your identity, not as it was, but as it is becoming— stronger, more self-aware, more tender than before.

This story began with disappearance. With confusion and collapse. But it ends with presence. With you, here. Still living. Still loving. Still trying. And not just trying to endure, but to enjoy. To reclaim your joy like it belongs to you, because it does.

You are not just a fugitive.

You are a survivor.

A witness.

A storyteller.

And this is not the end. This is where the next chapter begins, on your terms, in your voice, one good day at a time.

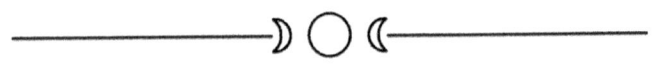

"The people who truly love you will not ask you to be easy. They will ask you to be real. And they will stay."

— *Jo Grey*

Printed in Dunstable, United Kingdom